Keto diet 2020

The ultimate beginner guide to a ketogenic diet. Learn how weight loss to regain your shape and live a healthy lifestyle

[Dr Steven Green]

Upon using the contents and information contained in this book, you agree to hold harmless the Author from and against any damages, costs, and expenses, including any legal fees potentially resulting from the application of any of the information provided by this book. This disclaimer applies to any loss, damages or injury caused by the use and application, whether directly or indirectly, of any advice or information presented, whether for breach of contract, tort, negligence, personal injury, criminal intent, or under any other cause of action.

You agree to accept all risks of using the information presented inside this book.

You agree that by continuing to read this book, where appropriate and/or necessary, you shall consult a professional (including but not limited to your doctor, attorney, or financial advisor or such other advisor as needed) before using any of the suggested remedies, techniques, or information in this book.

Table of Contents

INTRODUCTION 10

Chapter 1: What is Ketogenic Diet? 13

Chapter 2: What is Ketosis 16

Chapter 3: Keto Health Benefits 20

Chapter 4: Difference between Keto Diet and other diets 29

Chapter 5: Tips and Tricks to help you to gain your perfect shape 31

Maintaining Your Diet....................................31

Chapter 6: Workout on Keto Diet 35

Chapter 7: How to choose correct diet plan....39

Preparing Your Meals 39

Chapter 8: Shopping list................................41

Chapter 9: Breakfast Recipes 44

Asian Beef Short Ribs....................................44

Traditional fried Chicken................................45

Steamed Mahi-Mahi with Hummus..................46

Baked Herby Salmon 46

Chicken Coconut Curry..................................47

Greek Styled Lamb Chops..48

Chicken Puttanesca 49

Sun Dried Tomato and Artichoke Chicken 51

Zucchini Noodles with Sausages 51

Keto-Approved Beef Ragu.................................52

Bacon-Wrapped Roasted Asparagus 53

Simple Cod Piccata 54

Baked Salmon with Lemon and Thyme 55

Garlic Roasted Shrimp with Zucchini Pasta........55

Breakfast Blueberry Coconut Smoothie..............56

Vegan Chocolate Smoothie 57

Power Green Smoothie......................................57

Kiwi Coconut Smoothie 58

Mixed Nuts & Smoothie Breakfast.....................59

Superfood Red Smoothie 59

Coconut Shake with Avocado 60

Creamy Vanilla Keto Cappuccino.......................61

Golden Turmeric Latte with Nutmeg..................61

Almond Breakfast Smoothie..............................62

Quick Raspberry Vanilla Shake 63

Strawberry Chia Seed Pudding in Glass Jars.......63

Yummy Blue Cheese & Mushroom Omelet.........64

Chorizo Sausage Egg Cakes 65

Morning Herbed Eggs 65

Ham & Cheese Keto Sandwiches 66

Chapter 10: Lunch Recipes 68

Feta and Cauliflower Rice Stuffed Bell Peppers.... 68

Shrimp with Linguine 69

Mexican Cod Fillets 70

Simple Mushroom Chicken Mix 71

Squash Spaghetti with Bolognese Sauce 72

Healthy Halibut Fillets 72

Clean Salmon with Soy Sauce 73

Simple Salmon with Eggs 73

Easy Shrimp 74

Scallops with Mushroom Special 75

Delicious Creamy Crab Meat 75

Creamy Broccoli Stew 76

No Crust Tomato and Spinach Quiche............... 77

Peas Soup 78

Minty Lamb Stew 79

Ratatouille... 80

Steamed Artichokes....................................... 81

Creamed Savoy Cabbage................................ 82

Tilapia Delight.. 82

Spinach Tomatoes Mix 83

Spinach Almond Tortilla..84

Zucchini Noodles in Garlic and Parmesan Toss....85

Lemoned Broccoli 85

Beef and Cauliflower Stew 86

Chicken and Brussels Sprouts Stew.....................87

Cod and Shrimp Stew 87

Beef Meatballs Stew 88

Salmon Stew 89

Veggie Soup 90

Artichokes Cream 91

Leek Soup 92

Sage Chicken and Turkey Stew 92

Bell Peppers and Kale Soup 93

Tomato and Olives Stew...................................94

Creamy Brussels Sprouts Stew..........................95

Chapter 11: Snacks Recipes 96

Deviled Eggs...96

Cucumber Cups...97

Zucchini Sticks..98

Broccoli Tots..99

Cheesy Tomato Slices 100

Stuffed Tomatoes 101

Bacon Wrapped Asparagus...............................102

Mini Mushroom Pizzas 103

Jalapeño Poppers..103

Mozzarella Sticks 104

Cheese Balls 105

Parmesan Chicken Wings...................................106

Buffalo Chicken Bites 107

Mini Salmon Bites 109

Tilapia Strips...109

Coconut Shrimp 110

Bacon Wrapped Scallops...................................111

Chapter 12: Dinner Recipes......................113

Shrimp & Bacon Chowder 113

Creamy Salmon...114

Orange Chicken...115

Duck with Sauce..116

Pan-Seared Steak...117

Slow Cooked Beef Pot Roast...............................118

Stuffed Instant Pot Chicken Breasts 119

Slow Cooker Balsamic Roast Beef 120

Buffalo Turkey Balls 121

Stuffed Enchilada Peppers................................122

Keto Chicken Adobo 123

Basil Tomato Frittata....................................124

Chia Spinach Pancakes 125

Feta Kale Frittata 126

Protein Muffins 127

Healthy Waffles 127

Cheese Zucchini Eggplant 128

Coconut Kale Muffins...129

Blueberry Muffins 130

Coconut Bread 131

Pumpkin Muffins...132

Broccoli Nuggets...133

Cheesy Spinach Quiche 133

Vegetable Quiche 134

Coconut Porridge 135

Baked Eggplant Zucchini...136

Cheese Broccoli Bread 137

Shrimp Green Beans 137

Easy Asparagus Quiche 138

Olive Cheese Omelet..139

Cheese Almond Pancakes 140

Cauliflower Frittata 140

Chapter 13 : Dessert Recipes **142**

Keto Mocha Brownies 142

Keto Raspberry Cheesecake 143

Choco Cinnamon Cake.......................................145

Delicious Raspberry Muffins with Chocolate Topping
....146

Amazing Keto Almond Coffee Cups...................148

Keto Cherry Mousse...149

Chocolate Chip Pudding...................................150

Tasty Crumbled Lemon Muffin Parfait.............151

Sweet Potato & Cinnamon Patties...................153

Keto Coconut Bars...154

Chocolate Bounties..155

Lemon Cake...156

Choco Orange Muffins......................................158

Rum Cheesecake..159

CONCLUSION 162

INTRODUCTION

Health should be the first and foremost thing at the top of your list of priorities. There is always time to work hard and be successful, but if you don't pay your body its due attention, you cannot possibly enjoy all that you work hard for. Out of all the ailments that are caused due to the negligence of health, one of the most common is obesity or being overweight.

Over the years, there have been too many food choices for people to pick and eat. We don't check what we eat or how often and just let our body take it all in; however, there is a limit for your body to tolerate such things. Too much food will inadvertently lead to excessive weight gain. And most of these foods contain substances that are not healthy. At some point, you realize how your clothes don't fit or how lazy you feel all the time and need to take a thorough look at the state you have put your body in. This is when the regret kicks in and you try all the fad diets out there that claim to help you lose weight in a week.

This is not the approach you should take. Especially when it comes to health and losing weight, it is not about quick fixes. You could try starving for a week or only drinking liquids, and you might see the number on the scale go down a little, but what about later when you go back to your old food habits? Do you think the numbers will stay the same? Fad diets don't work most of the time and more often than not, they will harm your health rather than benefit you. Instead, why not try something that actually works?

In this book, you will read everything you need to know about the ketogenic diet. You might already have heard of it or this might be the first time you came across the keto diet concept. Here you will learn how you can include the ketogenic diet as a part of your lifestyle and how it will benefit you. It is not about starving yourself but giving your body the right kind of food in the right quantities. Unlike other fad diets, the keto diet will show you real results that will last over time. The book discusses in detail about getting started on the diet and following it in the right manner so you get optimal results.

A ketogenic diet will drastically reduce your daily carb intake and replace it with healthy fat. The reduction of carb helps the body to assume a state known as ketosis.

 In this condition, the body becomes extremely efficient and burns fat for energy. It also helps to transform fat into ketones in the liver, which results in supplying energy to the brain.

With a ketogenic diet, one can experience huge reductions in insulin levels and blood sugar. The increased number of ketones includes a number of health benefits.

A number of versions of the ketogenic diet are noted:

•   Standard ketogenic diet or SKD is a moderate-protein, low-carb, and high-fat diet, which contains 20% protein, 5% carbs, and 75% fat.

•   Targeted ketogenic diet or TKD includes carbs around workouts.

•   Cyclical ketogenic diet or CKD allows you to have higher carb refeeds like 5 intense ketogenic days followed by 2 high-carb days.

•   The high-protein ketogenic diet is almost like a standard ketogenic diet with the only exception of including more protein. The ratio stands at 60% fat, 5% carb, and 35% protein.

Cyclical and targeted ketogenic diets are more advanced and usually are given to athletes and bodybuilders.

A ketogenic diet is one of the effective ways to lose weight and decrease factors for disease such as high pressure and high blood sugar. It has been found out that people in a ketogenic diet have lost 2.2 times more weight than those in a calorie-restricted low-fat diet.

Apart from regular diseases, the ketogenic diet has also proved to be beneficial for several types of cancer and slow the growth of the tumor. It has also shown remarkable progress in people who have Alzheimer's disease; the diet has slowed the development of the disease.

Women suffering from PCOS or polycystic ovary syndrome have seen a remarkable decrease in their insulin levels. Once the insulin levels are decreased, one can see a remarkable improvement in the outbreak of acne.

Chapter 1: What is Ketogenic Diet?

By eating fewer carbs, you induce your body to the state of ketosis thus making it easier for the body to tap into the stored fat reserves it already has on hand. But getting yourself into the state of ketosis is never easy. Either you go on fasting for days or you cut down your carb intake to 50 grams daily, which is equivalent to around 5% of your total calories.

This can be achieved by changing your diet. Instead of taking in your usual diet, you can drive ketosis by eating more fat and protein. Your fat should be 60-75% of your daily calories while your protein intake should be 15-30% of your calories. This is equivalent to 1 large chicken breast and 5 small avocados each meal. Because fat is naturally filling, it will keep you full for a long time, so you will not feel the need to snack between meals.

The goal for the ketogenic diet is to get your body into the state of ketosis by breaking down fats into ketones as the primary source of fuel by eating the right amounts of food that support such metabolic pathway.

Is the Ketogenic Diet Really for You?

You have to remember that just like all other diet regimens, not everyone can follow a ketogenic diet. So, before you start this regimen, ask yourself if the ketogenic diet is really for you? Below are the things that you should consider to see if the ketogenic diet is for you.

•   **How long can I follow this diet?** The ketogenic diet is not like your usual fad diet only lasting for a few weeks. In order to see results, it will take you months or even a year. So, if you are someone who cannot follow its principles long-term, then this diet is not for you.

•   **Will the eating plan fit my food preference, budget needs, and culture?** If you follow a strict dietary guideline (veganism or vegetarianism) then you might need to tweak the ketogenic diet to fit your preferences. It may difficult, but not impossible. However, if you find it too much of a hassle to tweak the ketogenic meal plan to fit your preference, you might not enjoy this diet at all. •   **Do I have medical conditions that will put me at risk?** While the ketogenic diet has therapeutic effects to people who suffer from diabetes and cardiovascular diseases, it is not prescribed among people who suffer from kidney-related problems as the presence of protein and fats can be damaging to the kidneys.

The bottom line is that while the ketogenic diet is good for most people, it may not be advisable for some. So, before you ask yourself if this particular diet is for you, make sure that you seek advice from your nutritionist or physician.

How Exactly Does Ketogenic Work?

Since the carbohydrate intake for this particular diet is kept at a very low, carbs are practically absent thus the body is pushed to utilize other forms of energy in the form of fat.

In the absence of fat, the liver takes the fatty acids in the body then converts it into ketone bodies. You have to remember that the body just cannot take fat and use it in its raw form. It has to undergo different processes so that it can be utilized effectively by the body. This is the reason why it needs to convert it into ketone form. This process is called ketosis, and this is what the ketogenic diet is all about.

In a nutshell, there are three types of ketone bodies created during the break down of fatty acids and these include (1) acetoacetate, (2) beta-hydroxybutyric acid, and (3) acetone.

Before you can experience the many benefits of the ketogenic diet, it is important that you eat mostly fat. But how much fat is too much? When I first started, I had this misinformed idea that all I need to do is to eat all the fatty foods that I see. This was easy as pie, I said. And to tell you the truth, I see countless of dieters out there who make the same mistake that I did.

In order to succeed with the ketogenic diet, you don't need to eat a lot of fat. Rather, you need to smartly break down what you eat to 70-80% fat, 20-25% protein, and 5-10% carbohydrates.

You have to remember that the ratio varies depending on different people thus using an online calculator can greatly help! Make sure that you stick by your macros. The problem with most people is that they tend to eat more protein thinking that protein is always equivalent to fat. Well, not quite. Once you consume protein, the protein will be broken down into a process known as gluconeogenesis and it converts protein into carbs. So, you are back to square one.

To ensure that your body is constantly in the state of ketosis, you need to test the ketone levels in your body to know whether your body is still driving under this state or if you reverted back to your usual glucose-feeding metabolism.

There are several ways to test your body for the presence of ketones. Remember that when your body starts to burn off fats as its main energy source, ketones are spilled over into your blood and urine. And it is even present in you breathe! Since ketones are spilled all over the body, you can test either your urine or breath for its presence. You don't need to punch a tiny hole on your skin for blood testing.

Chapter 2: What is Ketosis

Ketosis is the metabolic state where your body uses fat as the primary source of fuel instead of sugar. The body can only transform into the state of ketosis if glycogen stored in your muscles are used up and blood sugar is low. The best way to achieve this is to follow a low-carb diet or fast until you experience symptoms of ketosis. Ketosis is hailed as an effective quick way to burn body fat and studies indicate that ketosis can positively impact our health in various ways.

How does ketosis work? Usually, your body is energized using sugar acquired from carbohydrates. However, if you extremely limit your carb intake, your body will force itself into reserved glucose, known as glycogen. Once glycogen is depleted, which typically takes 3 days, your liver will enter the process known as ketogenesis to utilize fat and produce ketone bodies. Ketone bodies are byproducts of burning fat in the body.

How to Start Ketosis

Most people eat a high carb diet which keeps them in a state of glycolysis, which means that your body runs on glucose for energy. When you're in this state your glucose will spike, causing your insulin to spike, after each meal. This promotes fat storage and blocks the release of fat from the adipose tissues (fat storage tissues).

However, with a low carb diet your body has to enter in to the state of ketosis. This is a metabolic state where your body breaks down fat and turns it into ketones. Your body then uses these ketones for fuel, and the ketones turn into your body's main source of energy. In the state of ketosis your body is constantly releasing fat to consume it. to enter into ketosis, you have to eat a low carb diet for a few days consecutively to tell your body that it will not be getting the usual glucose and force the switch.

Both amino acids that come from protein and fatty acids that come from fat are essential to your survival. Carbs are not essential, and you can live without them. While you do need some glucose to survive, your body will adjust to make that on its own. Most of the cells in your body can use ketones to survive. However, for cells that can only consume glucose such as the brain the liver adjusts. It takes glycerol from dietary fats and the liver makes it into glucose through the process of gluconeogenesis.

The goal of the ketogenic diet is to keep you in a state of ketosis without sacrificing your nutritional needs. Sadly, starting the ketogenic diet isn't an easy process. It takes your body time to be fully adapted to keto, which can vary from person to person. Some people take as little to four weeks but some people take as much as eight weeks to fully adapt, and that's only when you follow the rules regularly. If you break one of the rules of the diet, you're setting your body back to the starting line.

When your body is adapted to ketosis, glycogen decreases. This means your body will carry less water weight, the endurance for your muscles increases, and your energy levels increase. Luckily, when you are keto adapted, and you mess up and eat too many carbs it'll be easier to get back into ketosis the second time around. When you are fully adapted to ketosis, you're also able to eat up to fifty grams of carbs a day and not break it. So you won't have to say goodbye to all carbs forever. Moderation is the key.

The Best Tips to Get into Ketosis

When we eat high-carb foods (such as starchy vegetables and fruits, beans, legumes, and grains) our body produces high glucose levels. The human body actually uses glucose for energy i.e. fuel. When we eat low-carb foods (such as meat, fish, dairy products and eggs), our body uses stored fat instead of glucose and then, after 3 to 4 days, it gets into ketosis. It means that the keto diet works if you're in the state of ketosis. How do you know if you are in ketosis? Most common symptoms include increased levels of ketones in your urine, dry mouth, bad breath with a fruity smell, dizziness, appetite suppression, headaches, increased energy levels, cramps, constipation, fatigue, irritability, and insomnia. You can purchase ketone test strips that can help you test ketone levels and track your progress. Here are the best tips to get into ketosis, which is a natural state of the metabolic process.

1. Increase your healthy fat intake. Contrary to prevailing opinion, fats are actually god for you. Try to eat fatty fish twice a week, use extra-virgin olive oil in salad dressings, snack on nuts, add an avocado to your breakfast, take omega-3 fatty acid. However, make sure to stick to your calorie limit.

2. Try ancient practice of intermittent fasting. It can kickstart ketosis faster and help you maintain that state. You can eat during an 8-hour window or a 4-hour window. Many studies have proven that animals who have long-term caloric restriction may live longer. Other studies have shown that intermittent fasting may boost human metabolism, slow down aging, and produce antioxidants.

3. Variety is the key. Eat your favorite keto-friendly food. It's important to include a variety of foods to ensure you're getting all nutrients. In this collection, I tried to cover all food groups so It will help you sustain the diet without getting bored. The recipes are grouped into 9 categories: poultry, vegetables, beef, pork, seafood, eggs & dairy, vegetarian, snacks, and desserts.

4. Use MCT Oil. It can help you lose weight and boost energy levels. It may also help to lower blood sugar levels and bad cholesterol. Medium chain triglyceride oil goes directly to the liver, turning into ketone bodies. I like my morning coffee with MCT oil and coconut oil; if you do not like coffee, MCT keto smoothie can help you jump start your day, too.

5. Consume protein-rich foods. These building blocks can help prevent muscle loss and injuries, maintain healthy skin, and reduce appetite. Twenty percent of daily calories should come from protein in order to stay in ketosis.

6. Do not underestimate the importance of the physical activity. You can practice low-intensity cardio workouts such as jogging and cycling. According to experts, one of the most effective workouts for people on a keto diet is a strength training exercise (e.g. weightlifting). And last but not least, stay hydrated on the   keto-diet.

Chapter 3: Keto Health Benefits

The Keto diet is popular not only because you are able to lose weight fast but also because it has many other benefits. Changing your eating habits will affect your body in a positive way. Not only will you look good but your body will feel good, too! You will start noticing changes in your body within the first week or two of being on the diet. Eliminating the toxins you were used to ingesting will make a difference. The list below is not comprehensive by any means but will give you a good idea of what benefits that the Keto diet has to offer aside from the sought-out weight loss that the Keto diet is known for. Almost everyone will see significant improvements from the diet whether it be from the list below or from other things that have not been mentioned. Since we are all different and our bodies all react differently, you may experience things that others may or will not experience. The following list is what I have thought to be profound benefits that the Keto diet has to offer.

Nonalcoholic Fatty Liver Disease

Nonalcoholic fatty liver disease is a disease when your liver stores too much in its cells. The fat cells that the liver stores are not related to actual fat but to carbs. The livers transform the carbs into triglycerides and store them as fat. This disease affects people of all ages who are at risk of being overweight or obese, have high blood pressure, have type 2 diabetes to name a few. This disease could potentially have no sign or symptom but some people have reported fatigue and pain in their upper right abdomen, spider-like blood vessels, jaundice (the yellowing of the skin) and edema (swelling of the legs). Since the possible warning signs are linked to other ailments, there are often other tests that your doctor may have you take such as blood and imaging test.

Potential complications from this disease are the liver swelling. This swelling can cause scarring which could potentially lead to liver or even liver failure. There are no medications to help this condition as of yet but the Keto diet has helped countless people remove the carbs that their diets once had, therefore, lowering the triglycerides. The fat cells do not build up but instead, the liver uses it as energy. In some cases, people who have had scarring on their livers show a significant improvement because the body is essentially going through a rejuvenation process that will lead to a healthy you!

High Blood Sugar

We have sugar in our blood. The correct amounts are vital because sugar causes our body's cells and organs to obtain the energy we need to survive. If your body receives too much sugar, instead of having an abundance of energy you, you start to feel unwell. Your body cannot break down the as much of the overflow of sugar and this is why you start feeling the symptoms of high blood sugar. You feel drowsy, tired, have blurred vision, headaches, you have a hard time concentrating, tend to be thirsty, having to urinate quite often to name a few. These are short-term complications for having high blood sugar. Long-term complications can possibly include a heart attack or stroke, kidney failure and nerve problems. There are many causes of having high blood pressure. Your medical professional is able to diagnose long-term issues with high blood pressure as type 1 or 2 diabetes and in some cases gestational diabetes. Diabetes is caused when your body is unable to make insulin or there is not enough insulin in order to break down any sugar produced by carbs.

Gestational diabetes only occurs in women who are pregnant. Being on the Keto diet will help you be able to manage your diabetes by eliminating the carbs that are not able to be broken down by the insulin. You may also be able to reduce the medications you are prescribed. The lack of carbs in your system will make it easier on your body's functions.

Improved Digestion

Many of us have a problem with our digestive systems. From diarrhea, IBS (irritable bowel syndrome), constipation, and heartburn. We have all had at least three of these once in our lives. Constipation usually occurs when you are not eating enough fiber or not drinking enough water among other things. On the opposite end, there is diarrhea. This can be caused by multiple things as well as consuming artificial sweeteners, or certain additives. Acid reflux or heartburn is caused by stomach fluids backing up into your esophagus. Different types of foods can cause this back up especially if they are fatty or fried foods. Being overweight also has a high risk of heartburn. IBS or irritable bowel syndrome affects your large intestine. The symptoms for it are bloating, gas, cramping. Diarrhea or constipation. The triggers of IBS include but aren't limited to certain fatty foods i.e. deep-fried and carbonated drinks. Removing all the fired, greasy and carbonated drinks from your diet will help you improve your digestion. Everyone can benefit from the Keto diet because we all have experienced digestive problems at one time or another. The Keto diet helps you stay on track to avoid all these foods and stick to the healthy ones that will not cause all the above-stated issues.

Lowering Triglycerides

Triglycerides, as stated before, are a type of fat found in your body. If you have high triglycerides you are at risk for your arteries to harden which dramatically increases your risk of a stroke, heart attack or heart disease. Your medical professional has probably checked your levels at one point with a "lipid panel." This is how they diagnosis this. If you focus on what you eat and exercise, you will have a better chance of lowering them. Avoiding sugar and refined carbs can increase these levels. In addition, eating foods with Trans fats or hydrogenated oils or fats can increase levels as well. Focusing on healthier fats such as red meat and fish will help combat high levels. If you are prescribed medications for high triglycerides, the medication and an improvement in your diet should help reduce those dangerous high levels.

Depression

Depression is categorized as a mood disorder that causes a constant feeling of sadness. It also causes people to lose interest in things they once loved. This mood disorder is a constant in your life and you cannot one day wake up and be a happier you. Some symptoms of depression include hopelessness, anger, and frustration, being tired all the time, having no energy, trouble thinking, and anxiety feeling of guilt and sleep disturbances. There are still studies conducted on what exactly causes depression but so far, research has shown that what can lead to depression may be brain chemistry and how neurotransmitters react with other chemicals that should create mood stability.

Some other studies have shown that it might be an inherited trait. A blood relative might have passed down a gene with this particular trait that lacks the function to balance out your moods. Your body needs to be able to convert glutamate (a transmitter that your body has in order to get "messages" to the brain; you're welcome! I didn't know what this was either!) Into GABA (this is the body's main neurotransmitter). You need the right balance of both in order to have your brain function normally. When you are on a high carb diet, your brain isn't able to convert enough glutamate to GABA. This means that your body is suffering from neurotoxicity. Having your body goes into Ketosis, it seems to encourage the balance of both glutamate and GABA which alleviates the symptoms of depression.

Acne

Acne, as many of us know, is a skin condition that starts from adolescence during puberty and sometimes follows us into our adult life. The root cause of acne is when a pore in your skin becomes clogged, bacteria, excess of the androgens hormone, or excess oil production. There are different types of acne which include whiteheads, blackheads, and pimples (zits). They can appear on your face, forehead, chest upper back and shoulders. We know how slightly they can be and sometimes painful! There are many myths surrounded by what affects acne. Such as the makeup you wear, hygiene and eating greasy foods. One of the actual triggers that can lead to acne is your diet. Eating too many carbohydrate-rich foods. Eating all these carbs can alter your stomach bacteria because you are adding excess sugar to your bloodstream which can cause inflammation of the skin among other things. If you reduce your intake of these carbs, you reduce the risk of inflamed skin. You can also consume more fatty fish that are rich in omega-3, eat the lowest carb-filled vegetables and limit your dairy intake to maximize the benefit.

Heart Health

Keto can also benefit your heart health! Losing weight and can help you lessen the risk of heart disease. This is two for the price of one! Cardiovascular disease is actually an umbrella term that incorporates various issues that affect your health regarding blood vessels or heart problems. In this section, I will only be focusing on Coronary Artery Disease (CAD). This disease is when your heart is damaged by the buildup of plaque in the heart's major blood vessels. The buildup limits the blood flow to the heart and this will limit the flow of oxygen as well. Your doctor will typically run a lab test in order to diagnosis you. This disease is very common and affects approximately 3 million people across the United States. CAD can end up weakening the heart muscles which in turn can cause heart failure. Heart failure is when your heart cannot pump the blood the rest of your body needs. CAD can also cause heart arrhythmias. Heart arrhythmias are changes in the way your heartbeats. Instead of having a steady beat it is either beating too fast, too slow or irregularly. By reducing the intake of carbs, you are able to try and reduce or not add any more of the buildup of the fatty deposits that are associated with the CAD.

Brain Health

As mentioned at the beginning of this book, the Keto diet has been used to aid in the treat seizure disorders commonly known as epilepsy. Epilepsy is a central nervous system disorder that causes brain activity to become abnormal. There are different types of symptoms including twitching in the arms or possibly legs as well as staring out into nothingness for a short period of time with a blank stare. Once you have a seizure, your seizures typically tend to stay the same and nothing will change drastically. There are many causes of this disorder. A few are head trauma, brain conditions such as tumors or strokes, and injuries to the brain before birth such as lack of oxygen and developmental disorders. Your medical will review your symptoms and order a neurological exam which includes testing motor skills and mental focus as well as blood exams, EEGs, CT scans, MRI, PETs to name a few. Several studies have shown that the Keto diet has been linked to patients who have seen a reduction in the number of seizure episodes they have. Having the body go into the ketosis stage helps in altering your brain's metabolism in order to reduce the risk of having seizures. Many experts use the Keto diet as an aid to reduce seizures. Patients are still medicated but are still on the Keto diet to bring out the best outcome for the patient. Studies are being conducted for more brain conditions in hopes of either finding a cure or helping patients live a better life.

Migraines

Migraines are caused when nerve cells are overactive ad send out the incorrect signals to the nerves that are connected to your head and face. Sending these signals causes the chemical to be released and cause the blood vessels in the lining of your brain to swell. This is what causes the unbearable pain you experience when you have a migraine. There are a few triggers for migraines like changes in the weather, changes in your sleeping habits, skipping meals, caffeine, stress, and food. When you suffer from migraines you typically experience different "stages" before the actual onset of the migraine. The first stage is called the prodromal stage. The second stage is called the Aura stage. The third stage is called the Attack stage. The last stage is called the postdromal stage. In the first stage, you experience either high energy or being extremely depressed. You can also experience cravings, the need to urinate quite often and sleepiness. In the second stage, you start noticing changes in your vision, you may feel like you are on "pins and needles" and also may have difficulties with speaking or writing. In the third stage, the actual migraine begins. In this stage, you may have a migraine for, hopefully, just a few hours or it can last for several days. You are sensitive to light, you feel throbbing and it may only affect one side of your face or, in some cases, your whole face. Some people even have said they experience nausea and vomiting. In the last stage and when the migraine is over, you feel extremely tired and sometimes confused. A study done around 2009 showed that people who were on the Keto diet showed reduced signs of migraines. The researchers were first trying to have the patients lose weight to see if that would help them overall. The patients who were doing the Keto diet were the patients that had experienced the greatest reduction of migraines. They also had their non-overweight patients that suffer from migraines get on the Keto diet as well and they too had reduced amounts of migraines. Because of the low carbs in the Keto diet, researchers have found that it reduces the migraine causing inflammation of the blood vessels in the lining of your brain.

Muscle Mass and Performance

While you are on the Keto diet, you are able to increase your muscle mass as well. Carbs are not necessary to build the lean muscles some people are looking to create. In order to build muscle, you need to eat enough proteins, eating the calories in healthy fats and you need to weight train. You might gain muscle mass quicker if you are eating carbs but you need to remember that in eating carbs you will be eating the unhealthy fats that make you gain weight. If you are looking to maintain the lean muscles that you worked hard for, it is easier to maintain them on the Keto diet because you are losing fat and not your muscle mass. Studies have also shown that the Keto diet doesn't decrease your performance. Your body is just using a different way to energize itself. When you start the Keto diet, you will see a bit of a slowdown in your performance but this is expected because your body is going through a change that will take time to get adapted to. Once your body has now become accustomed to the way it is now converting fats into ketones, it will go back to where it once was performance-wise. You need to remember, though, to make sure that you are eating enough protein, calories, and training correctly, which are key. The Keto diet will hurt your body's performance nor will it hinder you from gaining or maintaining muscle mass.

The benefits listed here are just the tip of the iceberg when it comes to all the health benefits that the Keto diet has to offer. Enhanced weight loss is usually what people think of when they hear "Keto diet." Most are not aware of the vast benefits that are associated with the diet. A quick non-in depth review of other benefits include helping to manage your appetite, it is a way to maintain your weight because your body is always burning your fat, it can help aid in the treatment of metabolic syndrome, it aids in fighting different diseases which can include Parkinson's, TBI (Traumatic Brain Injury), and Alzheimer's to name just a few. Researchers are also starting to look into how the Keto diet may help with the possible removal of sugar consumption and replace it in hopes of killing off the cancer cells.

You will also feel more energized. Who doesn't want to feel this way!? Since your cutting the dreaded carbs, you will not be getting the effects of the sugar rushes that your body was used to and you will always have that steady source of energy and not the sporadic one that we all wish would last for days. You will see a significant change in your overall mood and memory. Since you are eliminating ingredients that are not natural, your body will only be processing foods that it should be therefore not sending out unhealthy toxins that affect your mood and memory. Wouldn't it be nice to remember where you placed your keys instead of looking for them for about ten minutes before you realize they are in your hands? No? Was that just me?

The Keto diet will also help with recovering faster from exercise. Deciding to add that extra five or ten pounds to your training regimen and dreading the next few days because of the achy and sore muscles will be a thing of the past. You will be able to recover faster because your body will not be as inflamed because of the reduction of carbs.

You will also be able to enjoy better sleep. Because you are reducing your daily intake of sugar, you are able to allow your body to completely rest. You will not be waking up randomly in the middle of the night. You already have a million and one things running through your head at night after a long day of life. You will be able to relax and notice this difference when you lay down and go to sleep when you reach the **6th** lamb instead of the **554th** lamb who, by now, has the name of Marty. You will experience uninterrupted sleep and rest through the night.

Although there are tremendous amounts of benefits, you should always reach out to your health professional.

I cannot stress this enough. Your health professional will be able to help you be able to make informed decisions about what is best for you. He or she knows what you have been diagnosed with and will know what actions need to be taken in order to assist you in living a healthier life. You may suffer any one of these specific aliments I have listed but your health professional will be able to pinpoint and customize what you need in order to be successful in treating whatever ailments you have. He or she has had their proper medical training and will be able to assist you in deciding what the best methods are to aid or cure your aliments.

Chapter 4: Difference between Keto Diet and other diets

When you go on the ketogenic diet, you are going to start with reducing the number of carbs that you are taking in. Instead of eating all those carbs, you are going to start eating more fats in your diet. Now, this does not mean that you are able to eat any fat that you would like and that you can spend all day eating out at a fast food restaurant. In fact, this would still be really against what you are allowed to do on this diet.

In order to understand just how effective the keto diet can be, it is important to understand how most "traditional diets function as well.

For the most part, a lot of the diet plans that you will see on the market are going to encourage eating high carbs and low fat. Some of them don't even care about the types of carbs that you are eating, they just want you to avoid fat at all cost. Fat is the enemy in all of this, fat is the reason that you are gaining and keeping on the weight.

There are a few issues with this. First, eating too many carbs can be bad for the body. When you consume a lot of carbs, especially the bad ones, you are providing a temporary surge of energy, but soon you are going to crash, feeling more tired than before and wanting to eat more to get that energy back. This is a bad cycle to get into because you will keep seeing wide fluctuations in your blood sugars, eat too many calories, and you can make yourself sick. Over time, you won't use up all the energy from the carbs and in addition to gaining weight, you will gain extra fat around the stomach and issues with diabetes.

The second issue with these diet plans is that your body needs fats. You do need to be careful with the type of fats that you are consuming (there are good fats and bad fats), but if you completely eliminate the fats that you are consuming, you are going to end up with a body that really is lacking in an important nutrient that it needs.

Because of these two reasons, the traditional American diet, as well as many of the other diet plans that you may be considering using for your own needs, is completely unhealthy for the whole body. You need something else, something that is going to help you to burn through the calories, lower your blood sugar levels, and finally get rid of that weight and that extra stomach fat that is bothering you now.

The keto difference: Unlike these diets, the keto diet cuts right to the heart of the matter and limits the number of carbohydrates you can consume in a single day to 15 net grams. Net grams can be calculated by taking the number of carbs in an item and subtracting the amount of fiber it contains. Then, once the body enters a state of ketosis it will be primed to use up all of its fat stores, trimming problem areas and preventing new ones from forming.

The main difference of the keto diet is that it is very effective on rapid weight loss to compare to any other diet. If you want to lose your weight you must follow the keto diet.

Keto diet is more carbohydrate restrictive diet compare to another diet like the Atkin diet.

Normally our body uses glucose (carbohydrates) as a primary source of energy but while you are on a keto diet your body will push into the state of ketosis in which your body breaks down fats from the liver for energy instead of glucose (carbohydrates).

Keto diet is not only just a diet plan it also helps to treat certain medical conditions like Alzheimer's, Parkinson's, high blood pressure, type-2 diabetes, heart disease and it also very effective on epilepsy conditions.

Chapter 5: Tips and Tricks to help you to gain your perfect shape

We already touched on some parts of this topic in the last part of the previous chapter. In this chapter, we will discuss more strategies and scenarios where your motivation to avoid eating and to lose weight will be put to the test.

Maintaining Your Diet

People usually eat more than their fair share when they haven't planned their food source for the day. Office workers are prone to this problem. They are usually absorbed in their jobs and they don't give a lot of thought on the sources of their foods. This makes them reliant on unhealthy food sources like preserved food products or fast food.

You can avoid these sources of foods by planning out your meals throughout the day. You will have a stronger chance of resisting temptations of food if you are not hungry most of the time. To do this, you should evenly space your meal throughout the day.

The ideal meal plan is to eat 6 small meals in your waking hours. Most adults eat 3 big meals and countless snacks in between. After eating one of their big meals, they will probably feel hungry again after 2 hours. Because it is not yet time for another big meal, they snack on the available food sources around them. For most people, the basis for their food choices is the taste. Tasty foods are usually high in fats and calories. You can avoid choosing these by creating a weekly meal plan.

Think tortoise and hare when you think of diets and losing weight – it really is slow and steady that wins. So to keep you motivated and inspired to carry on, have a look at these common techniques for motivation and ask yourself if they would work for you.

- Sticking motivational quotes to your mirror

Visual reminders are never a bad thing so ask yourself if putting some motivational quotes on sticky notes on your mirror would help you. You can actually stick these noes anywhere – the fridge, in your car, on every day, just as little reminders about what you are trying to achieve

- Weight loss jars

Visualization techniques are some of the best ways to keep yourself motivated. Get two jars, clear ones because you need to see what's inside them, and some colored pebbles or glass balls. Put one pebble or ball into one of the jars for eerie pound that you weigh and, for every pound you lose, take it out of that jar and put it in the other one. A quick glance is enough to tell you how well you are doing.

- Food Labeling

It's one thing to pack up your lunch and your snacks for the day but what if you are tempted to eat it all in one sitting? Putting labels on the containers with the time you are meant to eat it and how many calories are in it can help you with portion control

- Leave your workout gear out and ready for use

It can be difficult to walk past mat that's been left unrolled without getting down to a couple of crunches or a few yoga poses but you could go one step further. Leave a set of hand dumbbells in your bedroom, perhaps a resistance band or an exercise ball in the lounge and your running shoes by the front door as way of reminding you that exercise is important.

- Buy some of your clothes in the next size down

While it's always good to think about how you are going to lose the weight, it's also good to think about how you are going to look when you have lost it. So prepare yourself for your weigh-in and buy a few clothes that are the next size down. Hang them where you can see them when you wake up and when you go to sleep.

- Pin a "fat" photo to your fridge

Find the worst photograph of yourself you can and pin it to your fridge door. That way, whenever you get the temptation and head to the fridge, that's the first thing you see. That should be motivation enough to leave the candy in the fridge and pick up an apple instead.

- Share your food journal

Everyone tells you that, when you are trying to lose weight you should keep a journal of everything you eat. That's all well and good but it doesn't stop you from falling down. What might do is when you opt to share your food journal with someone else. You can either email it to a close friend or family member that you know is going to support you or you can go all out and publish it on your social media pages for all your friends to see.

- Dress in your workout gear first thing every day

Even if you are not intending to head out for a workout straight away, wearing the clothes is a great was of making sure that you will get out of that door and go for a un instead of finding an excuse not to.

- Lolly sticks

Write down all your fitness and diet goals on lolly sticks, for example, 25 crunches, walk 2 miles, etc., and put them all in a plastic cup. Pull one out and complete it and the put the lolly stick in another cup. Label the cups appropriately so you can see how much you have done and how much is left to do. As one cup begins to empty and the other starts to fill, you will find yourself even more motivated to keep going.

- Always have food with you

Diets do not have to be restrictive. In fact, those that are restrictive are the ones that you are more likely to kick into touch. Being on a diet isn't necessarily about cutting down on the amount you eat, it's about changing what you eat and going hungry is not a good motivator. Always have food with you – a couple of bits of fruit, a tub of chopped up carrots, peppers and celery, a low fat yoghurt. That way, when you get the munchies, you will not be tempted to head for the bakery and pick up a double chocolate chip muffin with a side order of chocolate chip cookies. You will have food there to eat, healthy snacks that will keep you full and satisfied, and keep the cravings at bay. Knowing that you are not about to go hungry and fall into temptation is motivation enough to keep going.

Chapter 6: Workout on Keto Diet

If you are not an athlete, the standard keto diet should be good enough for you. You can use exercise to improve your health and speed up the process of losing fat. This can be done with some simple regular cardio. You don't need to and shouldn't start practicing high-intensity sports that need sugar in your body. Just try a little jogging or running to increase your heart rate. The keto diet actually helps to improve performance in this kind of exercise. Your heart rate during the cardio session should be between 50% to 70% of your maximum heart rate. It can have many health benefits for you in the long run.

When you first start the keto diet, go for a slower pace. You can increase your speed or heart rate more in the next few weeks once your body is adapted to the keto diet. At this point, your body won't be dependent solely on carbs for energy during this type of exercise and will learn to utilize fat. For beginners who haven't exercised much before, try about 15 minutes of cardio in the first week. Increase this time by another 5 to 10 minutes every few days after that.

Soon you should be able to do at least 45 minutes of healthy cardio exercise every day. You can try cycling, running, circuit training, swimming, aerobics, etc. as your choice for this exercise. You might feel very tired when you first start out but your stamina and endurance will get much better if you keep at it. Cardio is a great way to speed up fat loss and improve the overall health of your body and especially your heart.

For Those Who Lift Weights

Just because you are on a diet does not mean that you cannot improve your strength or power and increase muscle mass. You can definitely do these in the keto diet. Your body doesn't require glucose for any activity that is less than 10 seconds long. Therefore, brief exertions on muscle by weightlifting will not be impaired by a ketogenic diet. As long as the sets are not longer than 10 seconds each, weightlifters can easily follow the keto diet and see an improvement in performance as well. The ideal program would have each exercise performed in five or less reps in five or lesser sets. This will help to increase strength as well as power within the ketogenic diet for weightlifters. Lower reps have been known to maximize muscle gain compared to higher reps; the appropriate volume is what is necessary.

Those who don't want to change their old programs can try carb supplements with their keto diet; however, carbs are not necessary to build muscle even though they prevent muscle breakdown. You can still gain muscle on a ketogenic diet as long as your protein and calorie intake is sufficient.

For Those Who Practice High-Intensity Sports Or Activities

The ketogenic diet can be beneficial for endurance athletes but not for those who play sports like soccer or basketball. It is useful for athletes who are trying to lose weight and get in shape, but performance-wise, at least in the initial stage, it will decrease the ability of the performer. People who play sports like golf can easily follow the ketogenic diet, but for sports like rugby and soccer, the body is dependent on the glycolytic pathway for energy. The keto diet will harm the performance of such sportspersons. Easily digestible carbohydrates are a better source of energy for these kinds of sports.

In case of boxing or wrestling, keto dieting helps to lose water weight. Athletes can also choose to follow the keto diet during off seasons when they don't have to perform and need to watch their weight more carefully. Hence, any sport that requires short bursts of energy is suited for a keto diet.

There are many supplements that athletes, sportsmen and anyone who exercises can use during a ketogenic diet.

- Beta-alanine is a supplement suitable for bodybuilders or high-intensity athletes who rely on the glycolytic pathway.
- Taurine is a supplement that has shown to improve exercise performance and decrease fatigue.

- Caffeine supplements help due to its stimulatory effect and increased cortisol levels.
- Exogenous ketones are a source of instant energy and recommended for endurance athletes or cardio training.
- MCT's or Medium Chain Triglycerides are saturated fat supplements, which are also good for endurance athletes and cardio trainers.
- Creatine is the perfect supplement for anyone who wants to increase muscle mass and strength and is ideal for weightlifters.
- Protein powders like casein, whey, collagen, etc. help to get the required protein intake according to an individual's needs.
- Alpha GPC is said to enhance growth hormone secretion, power output, etc and is ideal for weightlifters and athletes.
- Fish oil is a commonly recommended supplement, which helps to stimulate muscle protein synthesis and boosts the process of recovery. L-Citrulline is ideal for most athletes other than golfers or powerlifters because it reduces fatigue and improves endurance.

Depending on the purpose of the supplement, you can get any that you particularly need for your body.

The ultimate aim of any bodyweight workout is to increase your resistance and muscle strength. It is said quite often that muscles do not have a mind of their own, meaning they are dumb and can understand only two things. That is, stretching and tensing up. This is a good aspect because they will respond to any stimuli you shoot at them. This means that your muscles are not bothered by what kind of resistance you are using while working them. They do not recognize whether you are using a dumb bell, a barbell or your body weight. What this shows is that it is quite possible to develop great looking muscles without having to step into a gym.

Many people can bench press heavy loads but cannot do a few push-ups continuously. This is because the bench press exercise is comparatively a stable workout program that enables you to rest your entire body on a bench, thereby providing you with all the support you need to lift heavy weights. Another aspect is, when you bench press all that you are doing is coordinating the efforts of your chest muscles, triceps and shoulders since the parts of your body are in a resting position. Whereas, when you do a push up as part of a bodyweight workout, you are balancing your body above the floor. This requires you to work your lower back, abs, legs and rotator cuffs to stabilize every time you do a push-up. No wonder, a push up is much tougher than a bench press. Push-ups are a much better option than the bench press when burning calories.

Ever watch gymnasts train. Well, most of the times they train using their body weight and nothing else. Quite often we see that the gymnasts have better bodies and more strength than your regular gym going, bodybuilder or weightlifter. This is quite amazing since gymnastics does not involve pumping iron or lifting max weights. The gymnasts rely only on bodyweight workout alone. With a few years of regular training, you will find that most male gymnasts can bench press double their bodyweight the very first time they try it. This is another shining example which suggests that a bodyweight workout is far superior any day to pumping iron.

A bodyweight workout should be done at least three times a week. Make sure that you rest for a day before working out again. When exercising, ensure that you rest for thirty seconds between each set. Finally, a bodyweight workout does not require you to spend huge sums of money to enroll in a gym. It does not involve lifting of weights and pumping iron. All that is required of you is to give your body the desired workout to develop muscular strength.

Chapter 7: How to choose correct diet plan

Before the week begins, you should plan the types of food that you will eat throughout the week. By doing this, you will be able to plan what to buy from the grocery store and adjust the amount of calories that you consume according to your fitness goals. A person living a sedentary lifestyle will need 1800-2600 calories per day. Women and older people generally need lesser amounts. To know how many calories to consume for you to lose weight, you should write down a list of the foods that you eat every day for one week and calculate the corresponding amount of calories that you consume in each day. You could have a nutritionist do this for you if you are not sure how many calories each food type has. Or for detailed information on how calories work and how many daily calories you need, you can check out my book "Fitness Nutrition".

It is easy to decrease the amount of calories that you consume if you take away the unhealthy types of foods from your diet. You should be aware of the food types that are high in calories. If you eat these types of food, you will eat too many calories before becoming full. Some of these food types are chocolate, cheese, sugar-filled drinks, nuts and dried fruit. A handful of chocolates for example is equivalent to 2 cups of rice in calories.

Preparing Your Meals

Keep in mind that we are trying to avoid those instances where you need to rely on preserved and fast foods in your meals and snacks. To do this, you will need to prepare your own food each day. It is highly suggested to prepare your food for the whole day every morning. You should follow the daily prescribed amount of calories when preparing your meals. The next step is to divide the food that you prepare into six and place them into vacuum sealed containers to preserve their freshness.

The average person is awake for 16 hours a day. That means that you should eat your meals every 2 and a half to 3 hours. If you want to avoid eating before you sleep, you could modify the process by eating only five times a day. You will eat slightly bigger meals but the amount of calories that you take in will still be the same.

By following this plan, you will reduce the amount of calories that you take in at one time. Your body will have more time to digest the foods that you take in and by the time you eat your next meal, your body will have already digested the majority of the previous meal.

Because your meals are evenly spaced, you will not become hungry in between meals. This will lessen your unhealthy snacking and prevent you from relying on fast foods and high-calorie packaged foods. You will be satisfied most the time, which means that you will have stronger will power to resist offers of food.

Chapter 8: Shopping list

Before you go grocery shopping, make sure you have a detailed list of what to buy. Here are a list of foods that you should center your shopping list around. Go through the list and write down the foods that you like in order to produce your next trip to the store.

Foods that should be on your "Must Have" List

- Eggs: Organic whole eggs are best

- Poultry: turkey or chicken

- Fatty Fish: herring, mackerel, or salmon

- Meat: Grass-fed pork, beef, bison, and organ meats

- Full-Fat Dairy: Mozzarella, goat cheese, brie, cream cheese, and cheddar

- Seeds and Nuts: Almonds, walnuts, macadamia, pumpkin seeds, flaxseed, or peanuts.

- Nut Butter: Almond, peanuts, and cashews

- Healthy Fats: Olive oil, coconut oil, coconut butter, or sesame oil

- Non-Starchy Vegetables: Broccoli, greens, tomatoes, peppers, and mushrooms

- Avocados: Whole avocados are able to be added into any meal or as a snack

- Condiments: Pepper, salt, vinegar, fresh herbs, lemon juice, and other spices

Foods that should be consumed in small servings or not at all

- Baked Goods and Bread (white bread, wheat bread, cookies, crackers, rolls, and donuts)

- Sugary Foods and Sweets (ice cream, sugar, candy, syrups, coconut sugar, and agave syrup)

- Sweetened Beverages (Juice, soda, sports drinks, and sweetened teas)

- Pasta (any types of noodles)

- Grain Products and Grains (oats, rice, wheat, tortillas, and cereals)

- Starchy Vegetables (sweet potatoes, white potatoes, corn, butternut squash, pumpkin, and peas)

- Legumes and Beans (chickpeas, black beans, lentils, and kidney beans)

- Fruit (grapes, pineapples, grapes, and citrus)

• High Carb Sauces (sugary salad dressings, barbecue sauce, and other dipping sauces)

• Alcoholic Beverages (sugary mixed drinks and beer)

Food that should not be consumed at all

• Unhealthy Fats (shortening, margarine, and vegetable oils like corn or canola oil)

• Processed Foods (packaged foods, fast food, and processed meats like lunch meats or hot dogs)

• Diet Food Products (These contain preservatives, artificial coloring, and sweeteners like aspartame.)

Beverages that can be consumed

• Water (This should be on the top of your list. Hydration throughout the day is crucial for health, and will help you lose weight as well.)

• Sparkling Water (Sparkling water is a great way to replace soda in your diet.)

• Unsweetened Coffee (Use heavy cream in order to add flavor to your coffee.)

• Unsweetened Green Tea (This is a great way to provide a drink, and give you extra benefits.)

If you would like to add flavor to water, experiment with lemon-peel or fresh mint.

It should also be noted that even though most alcoholic beverages do not fit into this type of diet, you are able to have small amounts of vodka or tequila mixed with soda water on occasion.

Chapter 9: Breakfast Recipes

Asian Beef Short Ribs

Total time: 12 hours 10 minutes

Ingredients

- 2 pounds beef short ribs

- 1 cup water

- 1 onion, diced

- 1 tablespoon Szechuan peppercorns

- 2 tablespoons curry powder

- 3 tablespoons coconut aminos

- 6-pieces star anise

- 6 tablespoons sesame oil

- Salt and pepper to taste

Directions:

Place all ingredients except for the sesame oil in the Instant Pot.

Close the lid and make sure that the steam release valve is set to "Venting."

Press the "Slow Cook" button and adjust the cooking time to 12 hours.

Once cooked, drizzled with sesame oil.

Let it cool. Evenly divide into suggested servings and place in meal prep containers.

Traditional fried Chicken

Total time: 45 minutes

Ingredients:

- 2 large eggs

- 8 chicken pieces, skin on and bone in

- ¼ cup heavy cream

- ¼ cup water

- ½ cup parmesan cheese

- ½ tsp onion powder

- ¾ cup plain whey protein

- 1 cup crushed pork rinds

- 1 tbsp oat fiber

- 1 tsp seasoning

- 1/8 tsp coarse black pepper

Directions:

Mix all the dry ingredients in a Ziploc bag. Set aside.

In a separate bowl, mix together water, eggs and cream.

Toss the chicken pieces in the egg mixture.

Pick the meat and drop to the bowl of dry ingredients. Toss the bag to evenly coat the chicken. Set aside.

Heat a fryer that has ¾-inchese of oil in high heat.

Place the chicken in the hot oil and cook for 30 to 40 minutes until golden brown.

Let it cool. Evenly divide into suggested servings and place in meal prep containers.

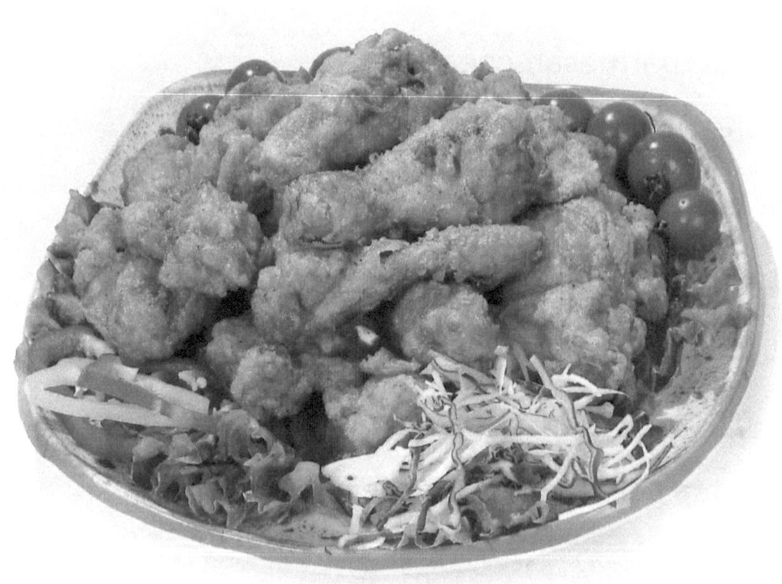

Steamed Mahi-Mahi with Hummus

Total time: 35 minutes

Ingredients:

- 2 filets Mahi Mahi fish

- Fresh coriander

- 2 tbsp lime, squeezed

- 2 tsp Philadelphia cheese

- 4 tbsp hummus

- Salt and pepper to taste

Directions:

Place Mahi mahi on a heat proof dish that fits in your steamer.

Season with pepper, salt, and lime.

Sprinkle cilantro on top. Securely cover top of dish with foil and place in steamer.

Steam for 30 minutes.

Let it cool. Evenly divide into suggested servings and place in meal prep containers.

Baked Herby Salmon

Total time: 20 minutes

Ingredients:

- 2 pounds salmon fillet

- ¼ tsp tarragon

- ¼ tsp thyme

- ½ cup coconut aminos

- ½ tsp basil

- ½ tsp ground ginger

- ½ tsp rosemary

- 1 tsp minced garlic

- 1 tsp dried oregano

- 4 tsp sesame oil

Directions:

In a Ziploc back, place the sesame oil, soy sauce and spices and shake thoroughly until well combined. Put the salmon pieces in the Ziploc bag. Refrigerate the salmon with the marinade for 4 hours.

Preheat the oven to 350ºF. Place the marinated salmon on a baking pan lined with aluminum foil.

Bake the marinated salmon for 15 minutes.

Let it cool. Evenly divide into suggested servings and place in meal prep containers.

Chicken Coconut Curry

Total time: 30 minutes

Ingredients:

- 1 ½ tsps curry powder

- ½ onion, sliced

- 1-lb chicken breast, cut into bite-sized pieces

- 1 tbsp avocado oil

- 2 tsps garlic, minced

- 1 tbsp coconut aminos

- 1 tbsp ginger, minced

- 1 ½ cups coconut milk

- 1/8 tsp salt

Directions:

On medium high heat, place a large nonstick saucepan and heat avocado oil.

Add chicken and stir fry for 9 minutes or until chicken is no longer pink. Transfer chicken to a plate leaving oil in pan.

Stir fry garlic, ginger, and onion for 3 minutes.

Season with curry, coconut aminos, and salt. Sauté for a minute.

Return chicken and sauté for 3 minutes.

Pour coconut milk, bring to a boil then low heat to a simmer. Simmer for 10 minutes.

Let it cool. Evenly divide into suggested servings and place in meal prep containers.

Greek Styled Lamb Chops

Total time: 10 minutes

Ingredients:

- 1 tbsp black pepper

- 1 tbsp dried oregano

- 1 tbsp minced garlic

- 2 tbsps lemon juice

- 2 tsp oil

- 2 tsp salt

- 8 pcs of lamb loin chops, around 4 oz

Directions:

In a big bowl or dish, combine the black pepper, salt, minced garlic, lemon juice and oregano. Then rub it equally on all sides of the lamb chops.

Then place a skillet on high heat. After a minute, coat skillet with the cooking spray and place the lamb chops. Sear lamb chops for a minute on each side.

Lower heat to medium, continue cooking lamb chops for 2-3 minutes per side or until desired doneness is reached.

Let it cool. Evenly divide into suggested servings and place in meal prep containers.

Chicken Puttanesca

Total time: 40 minutes

Ingredients:

- ¼ cup extra virgin olive oil

- ½ cup assorted Italian olives, pitted and coarsely chopped

- ½ tsp crushed red chili flakes

- 1 lb fresh tomatoes, diced

- 1 small red onion, diced

- 4 boneless chicken breasts

- 4 pieces boneless anchovy filets, coarsely chopped

- 4 pieces garlic cloves, minced

- Pepper and salt to taste

Directions:

On high heat, place an oven proof, large skillet.

Prepare chicken breasts by seasoning with pepper and salt and greasing with 2 tbsps extra virgin olive oil.

Sear chicken on hot skillet around 2 minutes per side or until golden brown on each side. When done searing, lower heat to medium-low, cover and cook until juices run clear. Around 6-8 minutes.

Remove from pan and transfer chicken to a platter.

On same skillet on medium heat, sauté chili flakes, capers, olives, anchovies, onions, garlic and remaining oil for 2 to 3 minutes.

Add tomatoes and season with pepper and salt. Increase heat to high and cook until you have a thick sauce, around 10 to 12 minutes.

Pour sauce on top of chicken.

Let it cool. Evenly divide into suggested servings and place in meal prep containers.

Sun Dried Tomato and Artichoke Chicken

Total time: 30 minutes

Ingredients:

- ¼ cup sun dried tomato pesto

- 1 14.5-oz can diced tomatoes with green peppers and onions

- 1 14-oz can artichoke hearts in water, drained and quartered

- 2 tsps olive oil

- 4 skinless, boneless chicken breast halves

- Pepper and salt to taste

Directions:

With pepper and salt, season all sides of chicken.

On medium high heat, place a large saucepan and heat oil until hot.

Add chicken and brown each side, around 5 minutes per side. Once done, transfer chicken to a plate.

In same pan, add tomatoes and stir fry for a minute. Scrape all sides of pan to incorporate browned bits.

Add artichokes and pesto. Cook and stir for a minute.

Return chicken to pan, cover and simmer for 10 minutes on medium heat.

Let it cool. Evenly divide into suggested servings and place in meal prep containers.

Zucchini Noodles with Sausages

Total time: 15 minutes

Ingredients:

- 2 cups of chicken sausages, sliced

- 2 large zucchinis

- 2 tablespoons coconut oil

- 4 garlic cloves, minced

- Salt and pepper to taste

Directions:

Make the zucchini noodles. You can do this with a mandolin, but you can also slice the zucchini into thin long strips using a knife.

In a skillet, heat up the oil over medium heat and sauté the garlic for three minutes while stirring constantly. Add the sausages and cook for another five minutes or until the sausages are cooked through.

Add the zucchini and season with salt and pepper to taste.

Let it cool. Evenly divide into suggested servings and place in meal prep containers.

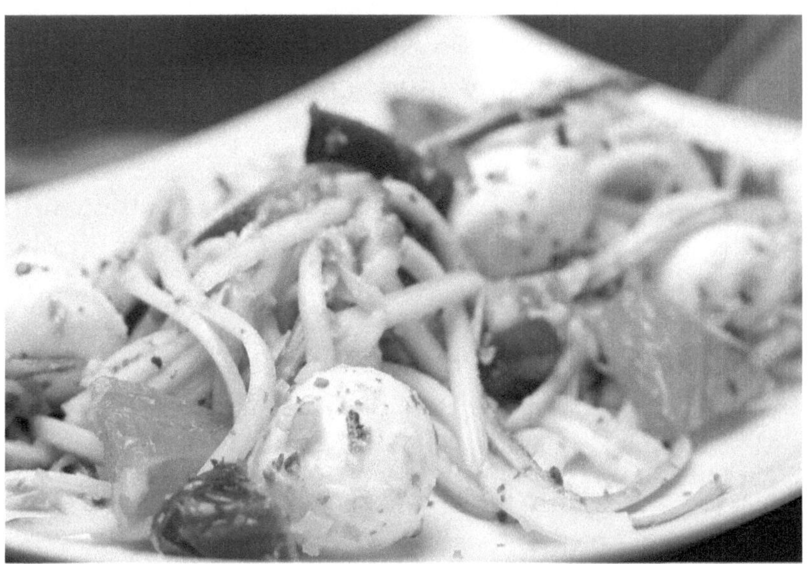

Keto-Approved Beef Ragu

Total time: 15 minutes

Ingredients:

- 1/4-pound ground beef

- 1 teaspoon salt

- 2 large zucchinis, cut into noodle strips

- 1 tablespoon ghee or butter

- 4 tablespoons fresh parsley, chopped

Directions:

Heat the ghee in a skillet under medium flame and cook the ground beef until thoroughly cooked, around 5 minutes.

Add the packaged pesto sauce and season with salt. Add the chopped parsley and cook for three more minutes. Set aside.

In the same saucepan, place the zucchini noodles and cook for five minutes. Turn off the heat then add the cooked meat. Mix well.

Let it cool. Evenly divide into suggested servings and place in meal prep containers.

Bacon-Wrapped Roasted Asparagus

Total time: 15 minutes

Ingredients:

- 16 asparagus spear, ends trimmed

- 16 pieces bacon

- 2 tablespoons extra-virgin olive oil

- Salt and pepper to taste

Directions:

Preheat the oven to 400⁰F.

Line a baking sheet with aluminum foil or parchment paper. Place the dry asparagus and place it on the baking sheet. Drizzle with olive oil and toss to coat. Add salt and pepper to taste.

Wrap each spear with the bacon. Bake for 10 more minutes.

Let it cool. Evenly divide into suggested servings and place in meal prep containers.

Simple Cod Piccata

Total time: 20 minutes

Ingredients:

- 1-pound cod fillets, patted dry

- ¼ cup capers, drained

- ½ teaspoon salt

- ¾ cup chicken stock

- 1/3 cup almond flour

- 2 tablespoon fresh parsley, chopped

- 2 tablespoon grapeseed oil

- 3 tablespoon extra-virgin oil

- 3 tablespoon lemon juice

Directions:

In a bowl, combine together the almond flour and salt.

Dredge the fish in the almond flour to coat. Set aside.

Heat a little bit of olive oil to coat a large skillet. Heat the skillet over medium high heat. Add grapeseed oil. Cook the cod for 3 minutes on each side to brown. Remove from the plate and place on a paper towel-lined plate.

In a saucepan, mix together the chicken stock, capers and lemon juice. Simmer to reduce the sauce to half. Add the remaining grapeseed oil.

Drizzle the fried cod with the sauce and sprinkle with parsley.

Let it cool. Evenly divide into suggested servings and place in meal prep containers.

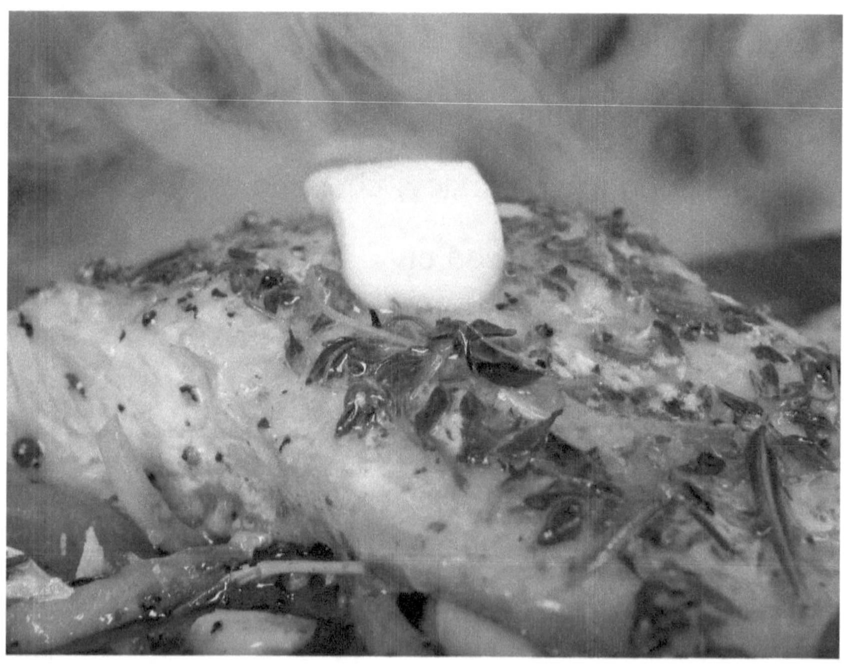

Baked Salmon with Lemon and Thyme

Total time: 30 minutes

Ingredients:

- 1-lb salmon fillet

- 1 lemon, sliced thinly

- 1 tablespoon capers, chopped

- 1 tablespoon fresh thyme, chopped

- Olive oil for drizzling

- Salt and pepper to taste

Directions:

Preheat the oven to 400^{0}F.

Line a baking sheet with parchment paper and place the salmon with skin side down.

Season the salmon with salt and pepper. Arrange the capers on top of the salmon and top with thyme and lemon slices.

Bake for 25 minutes.

Let it cool. Evenly divide into suggested servings and place in meal prep containers.

Garlic Roasted Shrimp with Zucchini Pasta

Total time: 20 minutes

Ingredients:

- 8 ounces shrimp, cleaned and deveined

- 1 lemon, zested and juiced

- 2 garlic cloves, minced

- 2 medium-sized zucchini, cut into thin strips or spaghetti noodles

- 2 tablespoon ghee, melted

- 2 tablespoon olive oil

- Salt and pepper to taste

Directions:

Preheat the oven to 400^{0}F.

In a mixing bowl, mix all ingredients except the zucchini noodles. Toss to coat the shrimp.

Bake for 10 minutes until the shrimp turn pink.

Add the zucchini pasta then toss. Turn oven off and just leave in oven for 5 minutes.

Remove from oven.

Let it cool. Evenly divide into suggested servings and place in meal prep containers.

Breakfast Blueberry Coconut Smoothie

Total time: 5 minutes

Ingredients

1 avocado, pitted and sliced

2 cups blueberries

1 cup coconut milk

6 tbsp coconut cream

2 tsp erythritol

2 tbsp coconut flakes

Directions

Combine the avocado slices, blueberries, coconut milk, coconut cream, erythritol, and ice cubes in a smoothie maker and blend until smooth. Pour the smoothie into drinking glasses, and serve sprinkled with coconut flakes.

Vegan Chocolate Smoothie

Total time: 10 minutes

Ingredients

¼ cup pumpkin seeds

¾ cup coconut milk

¼ cup water

1 ½ cups watercress

2 tsp vegan protein powder

1 tbsp chia seeds

1 tbsp unsweetened cocoa powder

Directions

In a blender, add all ingredients except for the chia seeds and process until creamy and uniform.Place into two glasses, dust with chia seeds and chill before serving.

Power Green Smoothie

Total time: 5 minutes

Ingredients

1 cup collard greens, chopped

3 stalks celery, chopped

1 ripe avocado, skinned, pitted, sliced

1 cup ice cubes

2 cups spinach, chopped

1 large cucumber, peeled and chopped

Chia seeds to garnish

Directions

Add the collard greens, celery, avocado, and ice cubes in a blender, and blend for 50 seconds. Add the spinach and cucumber, and process for another 40 seconds until smooth. Transfer the smoothie into glasses, garnish with chia seeds and serve right away.

Kiwi Coconut Smoothie

Total time: 3 minutes

Ingredients

2 kiwis, pulp scooped

1 tbsp xylitol

4 ice cubes

2 cups unsweetened coconut milk

1 cup coconut yogurt

Mint leaves to garnish

Directions

Process the kiwis, xylitol, coconut milk, yogurt, and ice cubes in a blender, until smooth, for about 3 minutes. Transfer to serving glasses, garnish with mint leaves, and serve.

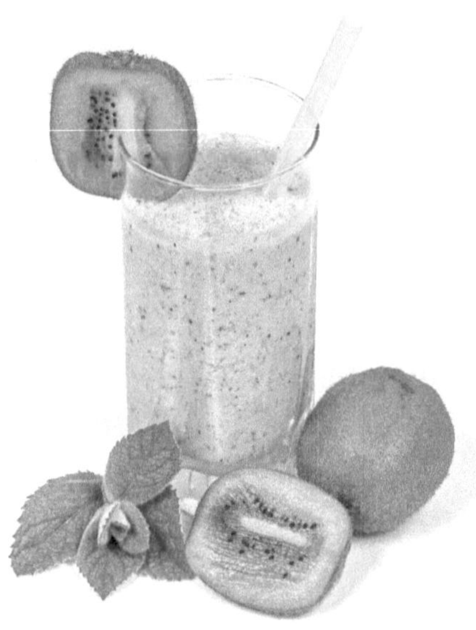

Mixed Nuts & Smoothie Breakfast

Total time: 5 minutes

Ingredients

3 cups buttermilk

2 tbsp peanut butter

1 tbsp unsweetened cocoa powder

2 tsp erythritol

1 cup mixed nuts, chopped for topping

Directions

Combine the buttermilk, peanut butter, cocoa powder, and erythritol in a smoothie maker; puree until smooth and well mixed.

Share the smoothie into breakfast bowls, top with mixed nuts, and serve.

Superfood Red Smoothie

Total time: 6 minutes

Ingredients

1 Granny Smith apple, peeled and chopped

1 cup strawberries + extra for garnishing

1 cup blueberries

2 small beets, peeled and chopped

2/3 cup ice cubes

½ lemon, juiced

2 cups almond milk

Directions

For the strawberries for garnishing, make a single deep cut on their sides, and set aside. In a smoothie maker, add the apples, strawberries, blueberries, beets, almond milk, and ice and blend the ingredients at high speed until nice and smooth, for about 75 seconds.

Add the lemon juice, and puree further for 30 seconds. Pour the drink into tall smoothie glasses, fix the reserved strawberries on each glass rim and serve with a straw.

Coconut Shake with Avocado

Total time: 4 minutes

Ingredients

3 cups coc

onut milk, chilled

1 avocado, pitted, peeled, sliced

2 tbsp erythritol

Coconut cream for topping

Directions

Combine the coconut milk, avocado, and erythritol, into the smoothie maker, and blend for 1 minute to smooth.

Pour the drink into serving glasses, lightly add some coconut cream on top of them, and garnish with mint leaves. Serve immediately.

Creamy Vanilla Keto Cappuccino

Total time: 6 minutes

Ingredients

2 cups unsweetened vanilla almond milk, chilled

1 tsp swerve sugar

½ tbsp powdered coffee

1 cup cottage cheese, cold

½ tsp vanilla bean paste

¼ tsp xanthan gum

Unsweetened chocolate shavings to garnish

Directions

In a blender, combine the almond milk, swerve sugar, cottage cheese, coffee, vanilla bean paste, and xanthan gum and process on high speed for 1 minute until smooth. Pour into tall shake glasses, sprinkle with chocolate shavings, and serve immediately.

Golden Turmeric Latte with Nutmeg

Total time: 7 minutes

Ingredients

2 cups almond milk

1/3 tsp cinnamon powder

½ cup brewed coffee

¼ tsp turmeric powder

1 tsp xylitol

Nutmeg powder to garnish

Directions

Add the almond milk, cinnamon powder, coffee, turmeric, and xylitol in the blender. Blend the ingredients at medium speed for 50 seconds and pour the mixture into a saucepan.

Over low heat, set the pan and heat through for 6 minutes, without boiling. Keep swirling the pan to prevent from boiling. Turn the heat off, and serve in latte cups, topped with nutmeg powder.

Almond Breakfast Smoothie

Total time: 4 minutes

Ingredients

2 cups almond milk

2 tbsp almond butter

½ cup Greek yogurt

1 tsp almond extract

1 tsp cinnamon

4 tbsp flax meal

30 drops of stevia

A handful of ice cubes

Directions

Put the yogurt, almond milk, almond butter, flax meal, almond extract, collagen peptides, and stevia to the bowl of a blender. Blend until uniform and smooth, for about 30 seconds.

Pour in smoothie glasses, add the ice cubes and sprinkle with cinnamon.

Quick Raspberry Vanilla Shake

Total time: 2 minutes

Ingredients

2 cups raspberries

2 tbsp erythritol

6 raspberries to garnish

½ cup cold unsweetened almond milk

2/3 tsp vanilla extract

½ cup heavy whipping cream

Directions

In a large blender, process the raspberries, milk, vanilla extract, whipping cream, and erythritol for 2 minutes; work in two batches if needed. The shake should be frosty.

Pour into glasses, stick in straws, garnish with raspberries and serve.

Strawberry Chia Seed Pudding in Glass Jars

Total time: 10 minutes

Ingredients

1 tsp vanilla extract

1 cup water

2 tbsp chia seeds

2 tbsp flax seed meal

4 tbsp almond meal

½ tsp granulated stevia

2 tbsp walnuts, chopped

4 mint leaves, chopped

½ cup strawberries, mashed

Directions

Place chia seeds, flaxseed meal, almond meal, strawberries, and granulated stevia in a bowl and pour over the water. Stir in vanilla. Refrigerate for at least 2 hours or overnight.

When the pudding is ready, spoon into glass jars, sprinkle with walnuts and mint serve warm.

Yummy Blue Cheese & Mushroom Omelet

Total time: 15 minutes

Ingredients

4 eggs, beaten

4 button mushrooms, sliced

Salt, to taste

1 tbsp olive oil

½ cup blue cheese, crumbled

1 tomato, thinly sliced

1 tbsp parsley, chopped

Directions

Set a pan over medium heat and warm the oil. Sauté the mushrooms for 5 minutes until tender; season with salt. Add in the eggs and cook as you swirl them around the pan using a spatula.

Cook eggs until partially set. Top with cheese; fold the omelet in half to enclose filling. Decorate with tomato and parsley and serve warm.

Chorizo Sausage Egg Cakes

Total time: 15 minutes

Ingredients

1 tsp butter, melted

4 eggs, beaten

Salt and black pepper, to taste

1 cup mozzarella cheese, grated

2 chorizo sausages, cooked and chopped

1 tbsp parsley, chopped

Directions

In a bowl, stir the eggs, sausages and cheese; season with salt and pepper. Add into greased with butter muffin cups, and bake in the oven for 8-10 minutes at 400 F. Sprinkle with parsley to serve.

Morning Herbed Eggs

Total time: 15 minutes

Ingredients

1 spring onion, finely chopped

2 tbsp butter

1 tsp fresh thyme

4 eggs

½ tsp sesame seeds

2 garlic cloves, minced

½ cup parsley, chopped

½ cup sage, chopped

¼ tsp cayenne pepper

Salt and black pepper, to taste

Directions

Melt butter in a non-stick skillet over medium heat. Add garlic, parsley, sage and thyme and cook for 30 seconds. Carefully crack the eggs into the skillet. Lower the heat and cook for 4-6 minutes.

Adjust the seasoning. When the eggs are just set, turn the heat off and transfer to a serving plate. Drizzle the cayenne pepper and sesame seeds on top of the egg. Top with spring onions and serve.

Ham & Cheese Keto Sandwiches

Total time: 15 minutes

Ingredients

4 eggs

½ tsp baking powder

5 tbsp butter, at room temperature

4 tbsp almond flour

2 tbsp psyllium husk powder

2 slices mozzarella cheese

2 slices smoked ham

Directions

To make the buns, whisk together almond flour, baking powder, 4 tbsp of butter, husk powder, and eggs in a bowl; mix until a dough forms. Place the batter in two oven-proof mugs, and microwave for 2 minutes or until firm. Remove, flip the buns over and cut in half.

Place a slice of mozzarella cheese and a slice of ham on one bun half and top with the other. Warm the remaining butter in a skillet. Add the sandwiches and grill until the cheese is melted and the buns are crispy.

Chapter 10: Lunch Recipes

Feta and Cauliflower Rice Stuffed Bell Peppers

Total time: 40 minutes

Ingredients

1 green Bell Pepper

1 red Bell Pepper

1 yellow Bell Pepper

½ cup Cauliflower rice

1 cup Feta cheese

1 Onion, sliced

2 Tomatoes, chopped

1 tbsp black Pepper

2-3 Garlic clove, minced

3 tbsp Lemon juice

3-4 green Olives, chopped

3-4 tbsp Olive oil

Yogurt Sauce:

1 clove Garlic, pressed

1 cup greek Yogurt

kosher Salt, to taste

juice from 1 Lemon

1 tbsp fresh Dill

Directions:

Grease the Instant Pot with olive oil. Make a cut at the top of the bell peppers near the stem. Place feta cheese, onion, olives, tomatoes, cauliflower rice, salt, black pepper, garlic powder, and lemon juice into a bowl; mix well.

Fill up the bell peppers with the feta mixture and insert in the Instant Pot. Set on Manual and cook on High pressure for 20 minutes. When the timer beeps, allow the pressure to release naturally for 5 minutes, then do a quick pressure release.

To prepare the yogurt sauce, combine garlic, yogurt, lemon juice, salt, and fresh dill.

Shrimp with Linguine

Total time: 25 minutes

Ingredients

1 lb Shrimp, cleaned

1 lb Linguine

1 tbsp Butter

½ cup white Wine

½ cup Parmesan cheese, shredded

2 Garlic cloves, minced

1 cup Parsley, chopped

Salt and Pepper, to taste

½ cup Coconut Cream, for garnish

½ Avocado, diced, for garnish

2 tbsp fresh Dill, for garnish

Directions:

Melt the butter on Sauté. Stir in linguine, garlic cloves and parsley. Cook for 4 minutes until aromatic. Add shrimp and white wine; season with salt and pepper, seal the lid.

Select Manual and cook for 5 minutes on High pressure. When ready, quick release the pressure. Unseal and remove the lid. Press Sauté, add the cheese and stir well until combined, for 30-40 seconds. Serve topped with the coconut cream, avocado, and dill.

Mexican Cod Fillets

Total time: 30 minutes

Ingredients

3 Cod fillets

1 Onion, sliced

2 cups Cabbage

Juice from 1 Lemon

1 Jalapeno Pepper

½ tsp Oregano

½ tsp Cumin powder

½ tsp Cayenne Pepper

2 tbsp Olive oil

Salt and black Pepper to taste

Directions:

Heat the oil on Sauté, and add onion, cabbage, lemon juice, jalapeño pepper, cayenne pepper, cumin powder and oregano, and stir to combine. Cook for 8-10 minutes.

Season with salt and black pepper. Arrange the cod fillets in the sauce, using a spoon to cover each piece with some of the sauce. Seal the lid and press Manual. Cook for 5 minutes on High pressure. When ready, do a quick release and serve.

Simple Mushroom Chicken Mix

Total time: 25 minutes

Ingredients

2 Tomatoes, chopped

½ lb Chicken, cooked and mashed

1 cup Broccoli, chopped

1 tbsp Butter

2 tbsp Mayonnaise

½ cup Mushroom soup

Salt and Pepper, to taste

1 Onion, sliced

Directions:

Once cooked, put the chicken into a bowl. In a separate bowl, mix the mayo, mushroom soup, tomatoes, onion, broccoli, and salt and pepper. Add the chicken.

Grease a round baking tray with butter. Put the mixture in a tray. Add 2 cups of water into the Instant Pot and place the trivet inside. Place the tray on top. Seal the lid, press Manual and cook for 14 minutes on High pressure. When ready, do a quick release.

Squash Spaghetti with Bolognese Sauce

Total time: 20 minutes

Ingredients

1 large Squash, cut into 2 and seed pulp removed

2 cups Water

Bolognese Sauce to serve

Directions

Place the trivet and add the water. Add in the squash, seal the lid, select Manual and cook on High Pressure for 8 minutes. Once ready, quickly release the pressure. Carefully remove the squash; use two forks to shred the inner skin. Serve with bolognese sauce.

Healthy Halibut Fillets

Total time: 20 minutes

Ingredients

2 Halibut fillets

1 tbsp Dill

1 tbsp Onion powder

1 cup Parsley, chopped

2 tbsp Paprika

1 tbsp Garlic powder

1 tbsp Lemon Pepper

2 tbsp Lemon juice

Directions:

Mix lemon juice, lemon pepper, garlic powder, and paprika, parsley, dill and onion powder in a bowl. Pour the mixture in the Instant pot and place the halibut fish over it.

Seal the lid, press Manual mode and cook for 10 minutes on High pressure. When ready, do a quick pressure release by setting the valve to venting.

Clean Salmon with Soy Sauce

Total time: 40 minutes

Ingredients

2 Salmon fillets

2 tbsp Avocado oil

2 tbsp Soy sauce

1 tbsp Garlic powder

1 tbsp fresh Dill to garnish

Salt and Pepper, to taste

Directions:

To make the marinade, thoroughly mix the soy sauce, avocado oil, salt, pepper and garlic powder into a bowl. Dip salmon in the mixture and place in the refrigerator for 20 minutes.

Transfer the contents to the Instant pot. Seal, set on Manual and cook for 10 minutes on high pressure. When ready, do a quick release. Serve topped with the fresh dill.

Simple Salmon with Eggs

Total time: 15 minutes

Ingredients

1 lb Salmon, cooked, mashed

2 Eggs, whisked

2 Onions, chopped

2 stalks celery, chopped

1 cup Parsley, chopped

1 tbsp Olive oil

Salt and Pepper, to taste

Directions:

Mix salmon, onion, celery, parsley, and salt and pepper, in a bowl. Form into 6 patties about 1 inch thick and dip them in the whisked eggs. Heat oil in the Instant pot on Sauté mode.

Add the patties to the pot and cook on both sides, for about 5 minutes and transfer to the plate. Allow to cool and serve.

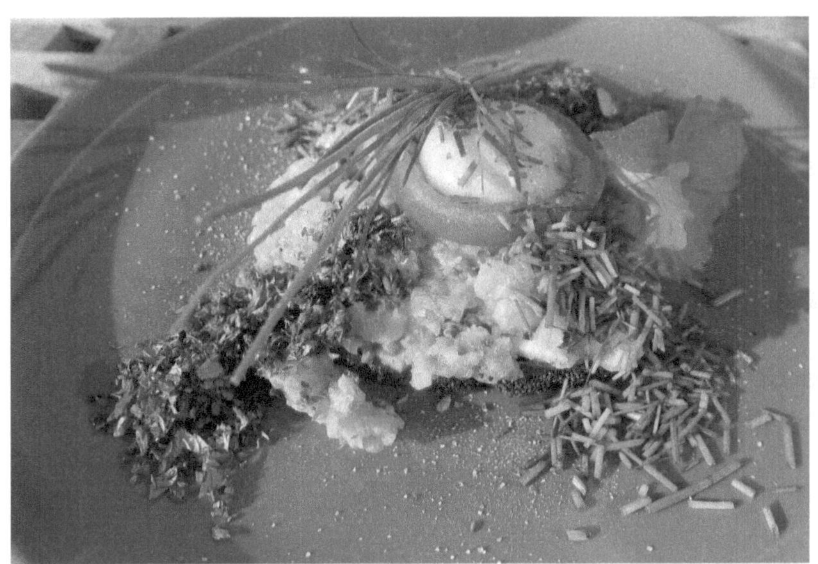

Easy Shrimp

Total time: 15 minutes

Ingredients

1 lb Shrimp, peeled and deveined

2 Garlic cloves, crushed

1 tbsp Butter.

A pinch of red Pepper

Salt and Pepper, to taste

1 cup Parsley, chopped

Directions:

Melt butter on Sauté mode. Add shrimp, garlic, red pepper, salt and pepper. Cook for 5 minutes, stirring occasionally the shrimp until pink. Serve topped with parsley.

Scallops with Mushroom Special

Total time: 30 minutes

Ingredients

1 lb Scallops

2 Onions, chopped

1 tbsp Butter

2 tbsp Olive oil

1 cup Mushrooms

Salt and Pepper, to taste

1 tbsp Lemon juice

½ cup Whipping Cream

1 tbsp chopped fresh Parsley

Directions:

Heat the oil on Sauté. Add onions, butter, mushrooms, salt and pepper. Cook for 3 to 5 minutes. Add the lemon juice and scallops. Lock the lid and set to Manual mode.

Cook for 15 minutes on High pressure. When ready, do a quick pressure release and carefully open the lid. Top with a drizzle of cream and fresh parsley.

Delicious Creamy Crab Meat

Total time: 20 minutes

Ingredients

1 lb Crab meat

½ cup Cream cheese

2 tbsp Mayonnaise

Salt and Pepper, to taste

1 tbsp Lemon juice

1 cup Cheddar cheese, shredded

Directions:

Mix mayo, cream cheese, salt and pepper, and lemon juice in a bowl. Add in crab meat and make small balls. Place the balls inside the pot. Seal the lid and press Manual.

Cook for 10 minutes on High pressure. When done, allow the pressure to release naturally for 10 minutes. Sprinkle the cheese over and serve!

Creamy Broccoli Stew

Total time: 55 minutes

Ingredients

1 cup Heavy Cream

3 oz. Parmesan cheese

1 cup Broccoli florets

2 Carrots, sliced

½ tbsp Garlic paste

¼ tbsp Turmeric powder

Salt and black Pepper, to taste

½ cup Vegetable broth

2 tbsp Butter

Directions:

Melt butter on Sauté mode. Add garlic and sauté for 30 seconds. Add broccoli and carrots, and cook until soft, for 2-3 minutes. Season with salt and pepper.

Stir in the vegetable broth and seal the lid. Cook on Meat/Stew mode for 40 minutes. When ready, do a quick pressure release. Stir in the heavy cream.

No Crust Tomato and Spinach Quiche

Total time: 45 minutes

Ingredients

14 large Eggs

1 cup Full Milk

Salt to taste

Ground Black Pepper to taste

4 cups fresh Baby Spinach, chopped

3 Tomatoes, diced

3 Scallions, sliced

2 Tomato, sliced into firm rings

½ cup Parmesan Cheese, shredded

Water for boiling

Directions

Place the trivet in the pot and pour in 1 ½ cups of water. Break the eggs into a bowl, add salt, pepper, and milk and whisk it. Share the diced tomatoes, spinach and scallions into 3 ramekins, gently stir, and arrange 3 slices of tomatoes on top in each ramekin.

Sprinkle with Parmesan cheese. Gently place the ramekins in the pot, and seal the lid. Select Manual and cook on High Pressure for 20 minutes. Once ready, quickly release the pressure.

Carefully remove the ramekins and use a paper towel to tap soak any water from the steam that sits on the quiche. Brown the top of the quiche with a fire torch.

Peas Soup

Total time: 20 minutes

Ingredients

1 white onion, chopped

1 tablespoon olive oil

1 quart veggie stock

2 eggs

3 tablespoons lemon juice

2 cups peas

2 tablespoons parmesan, grated

Salt and black pepper to the taste

Directions:

Heat up a pot with the oil over medium-high heat, add the onion and sauté for 4 minutes.

Add the rest of the ingredients except the eggs, bring to a simmer and cook for 4 minutes.

Add whisked eggs, stir the soup, cook for 2 minutes more, divide into bowls and serve.

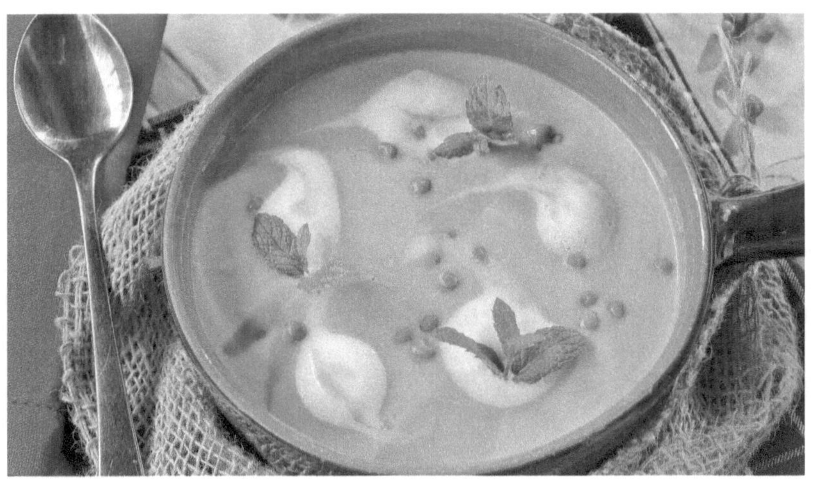

Minty Lamb Stew

Total time: 1 hour 55 minutes

Ingredients

3 cups orange juice

½ cup mint, chopped

Salt and black pepper to the taste

2 pounds lamb shoulder, boneless and cubed

3 tablespoons olive oil

1 carrot, chopped

1 yellow onion, chopped

1 celery rib, chopped

1 tablespoon ginger, grated

28 ounces canned tomatoes, crushed

1 tablespoon garlic, minced

1 cup apricots, dried and halved

½ cup mint, chopped

15 ounces canned chickpeas, drained

6 tablespoons Greek yogurt

Directions:

Heat up a pot with 2 tablespoons oil over medium-high heat, add the meat and brown for 5 minutes.

Add the carrot, onion, celery, garlic and the ginger, stir and sauté for 5 minutes more.

Add the rest of the ingredients except the yogurt, bring to a simmer and cook over medium heat for 1 hour and 30 minutes.

Divide the stew into bowls, top each serving with the yogurt and serve.

Ratatouille

Total time: 30 minutes

Ingredients

1 cup Water

3 tbsp Olive oil

2 Zucchinis, sliced in rings

2 Eggplants, sliced in rings

3 large Tomatoes, sliced in thick rings

1 medium Red Onion, sliced in thin rings

3 cloves Garlic, minced

2 sprigs Fresh Thyme

Salt to taste

Black Pepper to taste

4 tsp Plain Vinegar

Directions

Place all veggies in a bowl, sprinkle with salt and pepper; toss. Line foil in a spring form tin and arrange 1 slice each of the vegetables in, one after the other in a tight circular arrangement.

Fill the entire tin. Sprinkle the garlic over, some more black pepper and salt, and arrange the thyme sprigs on top. Drizzle olive oil and vinegar over the veggies.

Place a trivet to fit in the Instant Pot, pour the water in and place the veggies on the trivet. Seal the lid, secure the pressure valve and select Manual mode on High Pressure for 6 minutes. Once ready, quickly release the pressure. Carefully remove the tin and serve ratatouille.

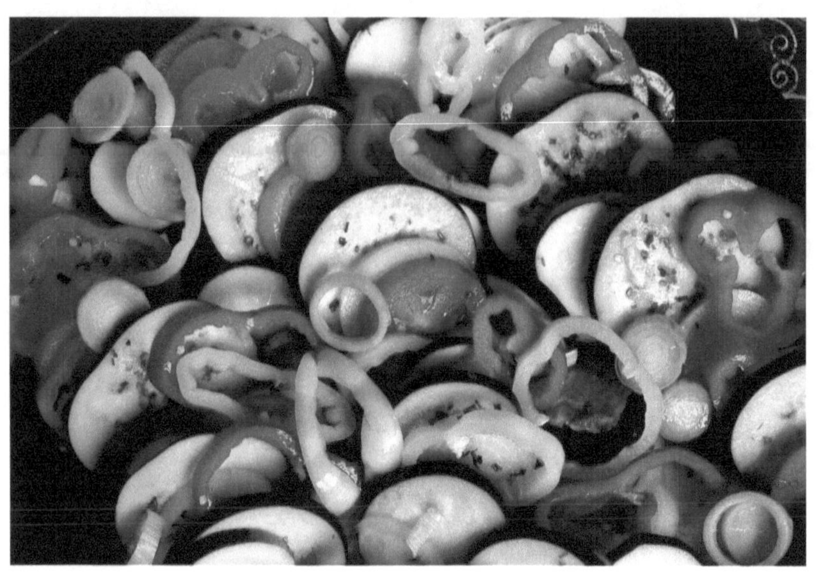

Steamed Artichokes

Total time: 35 minutes

Ingredients

2 medium Artichokes

3 Lemon Wedges (for cooking and serving)

1 ½ cup Water

Directions

Clean the artichokes by removing all dead leaves, the stem, and top third of it. Rub the top of the artichokes with the lemon. Set aside. Place a trivet to fit in the Instant Pot, pour in water.

Place the artichokes on the trivet, seal the lid. Select Manual mode on High Pressure for 9 minutes. Once the timer ends, keep the pressure valve for 10 minutes; then quickly release the remaining pressure. Remove artichokes and serve with garlic mayo and lemon wedges.

Creamed Savoy Cabbage

Total time: 30 minutes

Ingredients

2 medium Savoy Cabbages, finely chopped

2 small Onions, chopped

2 cups Bacon, chopped

2 ½ cups Mixed Bone Broth, see recipe above

¼ tsp Mace

2 cups Coconut Milk

1 Bay Leaf

Salt to taste

3 tbsp Chopped Parsley

Directions

Set on Sauté. Add the bacon crumbles and onions; cook until crispy. Add bone broth and scrape the bottom of the pot. Stir in bay leaf and cabbage. Cut out some parchment paper and cover the cabbage with it.

Seal the lid, select Manual mode and cook on High Pressure for 4 minutes. Once ready, press Cancel and quickly release the pressure. Select Sauteé, stir in the milk and nutmeg. Simmer for 5 minutes, add the parsley.

Tilapia Delight

Total time: 30 minutes

Ingredients

4 Tilapia fillets

4 tbsp Lemon juice

2 tbsp Butter

2 Garlic cloves

½ cup Parsley

Salt and Pepper, to taste

Directions:

Melt butter on Sauté, and add garlic cloves, parsley. Season with salt and pepper; stir well. Cook for 2 to 3 minutes. Then, add tilapia and lemon juice and stir well.

Seal the lid and set on Manual mode. Cook for 10 minutes on High pressure. When the timer beeps, allow the pressure to release naturally, for 5 minutes.

Spinach Tomatoes Mix

Total time: 20 minutes

Ingredients

2 tbsp Butter

1 Onion, chopped

2 cloves Garlic, minced

1 tbsp Cumin powder

1 tbsp Paprika

2 Tomatoes, chopped

2 cups Vegetable broth

1 small bunch of Spinach, chopped

Cilantro for garnishing

Directions:

Melt the butter on Sauté mode. Add onion, garlic, and cumin powder, paprika, and vegetable broth; stir well. Add in tomatoes and spinach. Seal the lid, press Manual and cook on High pressure for 10 minutes. When ready, do a quick pressure release.

Spinach Almond Tortilla

Total time: 25 minutes

Ingredients

1 cup Almond flour + extra for dusting

1 cup Spinach, chopped

¼ tbsp Chili flakes

¼ cup Mushrooms, sliced

½ tbsp Salt

2 tbsp Olive oil

Directions:

In a bowl, combine flour, mushrooms, spinach, salt, and flakes; mix well. Add ¼ cup of water and make a thick batter. Roll out the batter until is thin. Heat oil on Sauté mode.

Cook the tortilla for 5 minutes until golden brown. Serve with cilantro sauce and enjoy.

Zucchini Noodles in Garlic and Parmesan Toss

Total time: 30 minutes

Ingredients

3 large Zucchinis, spiralized

2 tbsp Olive oil

3 cloves Garlic, minced

1 Lemon, zested and juiced

Salt to taste

Black Pepper to taste

5 Mint Leaves, chopped

6 tbsp Parmesan Cheese, grated

Directions

Set on Sauté. Heat the oil, and add lemon zest, garlic, and salt. Stir and cook for 30 seconds. Add zucchini and pour lemon juice over. Coat the noodles quickly but gently with the oil.

Cook for 10 seconds, press Cancel. Sprinkle the mint leaves and cheese over and toss gently.

Lemoned Broccoli

Total time: 25 minutes

Ingredients

1 lb Broccoli, cut in biteable sizes

3 Lemon Slices

¼ cup Water

Salt to taste

Pepper to taste

Directions

Pour the water into the Instant Pot. Add the broccoli and sprinkle with lemon juice, pepper, and salt. Seal the lid, secure the pressure valve, and Manual in Low Pressure mode for 3 minutes. Once ready, quickly release the pressure. Drain the broccoli and serve as a side dish.

Beef and Cauliflower Stew

Total time: 35 minutes

Ingredients

1 tablespoon olive oil

2 shallots, chopped

A pinch of salt and black pepper

1 pound beef stew meat, cubed

15 ounces canned tomatoes, chopped

5 cups chicken stock

1 tablespoon cilantro, chopped

Directions:

Set your instant pot on Sauté mode, add the oil, heat it up, add the shallot and the meat and brown for 5 minutes.

Add the rest of the ingredients, put the lid on and cook on High for 20 minutes..

Release the pressure naturally for 10 minutes, divide the stew into bowls and serve.

Chicken and Brussels Sprouts Stew

Total time: 35 minutes

Ingredients

1 tablespoon avocado oil

2 scallions, chopped

1 pound chicken breasts, skinless, boneless and cubed

½ pound Brussels sprouts, halved

1 teaspoon basil, chopped

1 and ½ cups chicken stock

A pinch of salt and black pepper

1 tablespoon tomato paste

Directions:

Set your instant pot on Sauté mode, add the oil, heat it up, add the scallions and the chicken and brown for 5 minutes.

Add the remaining ingredients, put the lid on and cook on High for 20 minutes.

Release the pressure naturally for 10 minutes, divide the stew into bowls and serve.

Cod and Shrimp Stew

Total time: 19 minutes

Ingredients

1 and ½ pounds shrimp, peeled and deveined

1 and ½ pounds cod fillets, boneless, skinless and cubed

20 ounces canned tomatoes, chopped

3 garlic cloves, minced

2 tablespoons parsley, chopped

2 cups veggie stock

1 tablespoon basil, dried

A pinch of salt and black pepper

Directions:

In your instant pot, mix the shrimp with the cod and the rest of the ingredients, put the lid on and cook on High for 14 minutes.

Release the pressure fast for 5 minutes, divide the stew into bowls and serve.

Beef Meatballs Stew

Total time: 25 minutes

Ingredients

1 and ½ pounds beef meat, ground

1 egg

2 tablespoons cilantro, chopped

2 garlic cloves, minced

A pinch of salt and black pepper

¾ cup beef stock

½ cup tomato passata

½ teaspoon sweet paprika

2 tablespoons olive oil

1 tablespoon parsley, chopped

Directions:

In a bowl, mix the beef with the egg, salt, pepper, garlic and the cilantro, stir and shape medium meatballs out of this mix.

Set the instant pot on Sauté mode, add the oil, heat it up, add the meatballs and brown for 2 minutes on each side.

Add the rest of the ingredients, put the lid on and cook on High for 10 minutes.

Release the pressure naturally for 10 minutes, divide the mix between plates and serve.

Salmon Stew

Total time: 25 minutes

Ingredients

4 salmon fillets, boneless and cubed

2 cups chicken stock

2 tablespoons olive oil

2 shallots, chopped

2 tomatoes, cubed

1 tablespoon sweet paprika

½ teaspoon chili powder

1 zucchini, chopped

1 eggplant, chopped

A pinch of salt and black **pepper**

Directions:

Set the instant pot on Sauté mode, add the oil, heat it up, add the shallots and cook for 2 minutes.

Add the salmon and the rest of the ingredients, put the lid on and cook on High for 13 minutes.

Release the pressure naturally for 10 minutes, divide the stew into bowls and serve.

Veggie Soup

Total time: 25 minutes

Ingredients

1 tablespoon avocado oil

1 celery stalk, chopped

2 tomatoes, chopped

1 shallot, chopped

1 zucchini, chopped

2 garlic cloves, minced

6 cups chicken stock

A pinch of salt and black pepper

1 teaspoon basil, dried

2 cups kale, chopped

2 tablespoons basil, chopped

Directions:

Set your instant pot on Sauté mode, add oil, heat it up, add the shallot and the garlic and sauté for 2 minutes.

Add the rest of the ingredients except the basil, put the lid on and cook on High for 13 minutes.

Release the pressure naturally for 10 minutes, ladle into bowls and serve with the basil sprinkled on top.

Artichokes Cream

Total time: 25 minutes

Ingredients

2 cups artichoke hearts, chopped

3 tablespoons ghee

6 cups chicken stock

1 shallot, chopped

¼ teaspoon lime juice

1 teaspoon rosemary, dried

½ cup coconut cream

A pinch of salt and black pepper

Directions:

Set your instant pot on Sauté mode, add the ghee, heat it up, add the shallot and cook for 2 minutes.

Add the rest of the ingredients, put the lid on and cook on High for 13 minutes.

Release the pressure naturally for 10 minutes, blend the soup using an immersion blender, ladle into bowls and serve.

Leek Soup

Total time: 25 minutes

Ingredients

4 cups chicken stock

2 leeks, chopped

1 tablespoon olive oil

1 shallot, minced

1 tablespoon sweet paprika

1 tablespoon tomato paste

A pinch of salt and black pepper

1 tablespoon cilantro, chopped

Directions:

Set the instant pot on Sauté mode, add the oil, heat it up, add the shallot and the leeks and sauté for 2 minutes.

Add the rest of the ingredients, put the lid on and cook on High for 13 minutes.

Release the pressure naturally for 10 minutes, ladle the soup into bowls and serve.

Sage Chicken and Turkey Stew

Total time: 35 minutes

Ingredients

½ pound turkey breast, skinless, boneless and cubed

½ pound chicken breast, skinless, boneless and cubed

1 tablespoon sage, chopped

1 teaspoon olive oil

¼ pound tomatoes, cubed

1 shallot, chopped

A pinch of salt and black pepper

2 tablespoons tomato paste

2 and ½ cups chicken stock

1 tablespoon cilantro, chopped

Directions:

Set your instant pot on Sauté mode, add oil, heat it up, add the turkey, chicken and the shallots, and brown for 5 minutes.

Add the rest of the ingredients except the cilantro, put the lid on and cook on High for 20 minutes.

Release the pressure naturally for 10 minutes, divide the stew into bowls, sprinkle the cilantro on top and **serve.**

Bell Peppers and Kale Soup

Total time: 25 minutes

Ingredients

4 red bell peppers, deseeded and roughly chopped

½ pound kale, torn

A pinch of salt and black pepper

1 cup tomato passata

4 cups chicken stock

1 tablespoon cilantro, chopped

Directions:

In your instant pot, mix the bell peppers with the kale and the rest of the ingredients, put the lid on and cook on High for 15 minutes.

Release the pressure naturally for 10 minutes, ladle the soup into bowls and serve.

Tomato and Olives Stew

Total time: 20 minutes

Ingredients

1 pound tomatoes, cubed

1 tablespoon olive oil

A pinch of salt and black pepper

1 cup kalamata olives, pitted

1 teaspoon thyme, dried

1 cup chicken stock

1 tablespoon oregano, chopped

Directions:

Set your instant pot on Sauté mode, add the oil, heat it up, add the tomatoes and cook them for 2 minutes.

Add the rest of the ingredients except the oregano, put the lid on and cook on High for 15 minutes

Release the pressure fast for 5 minutes, add the oregano, stir, divide the stew into bowls and serve right away.

Creamy Brussels Sprouts Stew

Total time: 30 minutes

Ingredients

1 tablespoon olive oil

2 shallots, chopped

1 pound Brussels sprouts, halved

A pinch of salt and black pepper

1 cup chicken stock

1 cup coconut cream

1 tablespoon chives, chopped

Directions:

Set your instant pot on Sauté mode, add the oil, heat it up, add the shallots and sauté for 5 minutes.

Add the rest of the ingredients except the chives, put the lid on and cook on High for 20 minutes.

Release the pressure fast for 5 minutes, add the chives, stir the stew, divide it into bowls and serve.

Chapter 11: Snacks Recipes

Deviled Eggs

 Total time: 20 minutes

Ingredients

6 large organic eggs

¼ cup plain Greek yogurt

Salt, as required

3 tablespoons scallions, finely chopped

1 tablespoon Dijon mustard

Cayenne pepper, to taste

1 tablespoon chives, minced

Directions

In a pan of water, add the eggs and heat over high heat and bring to a boil.

Cover the pan and remove from heat.

Set the pan aside, covered for about 10-12 minutes.

Drain the eggs and set aside to cool completely.

Peel the eggs and with a sharp knife, slice them in half vertically.

Scoop out the yolks.

In a blender, add the egg yolks, yogurt, and salt and pulse until smooth.

Transfer the yogurt mixture into a bowl.

Add the scallion and mustard and stir to combine.

With a spoon, place the yogurt mixture evenly in each egg half.

Sprinkle with cayenne pepper and serve with the garnishing of chives.

Cucumber Cups

Total time: 20 minutes

Ingredients

8 ounces cooked salmon, very finely chopped

¼ cup coconut cream

1 tablespoon shallots, minced

1 tablespoon fresh chives, minced

¼ teaspoon smoked paprika

Salt and ground black pepper, as required

1 English cucumber, peeled and cut crosswise into ¾-inch thick slices

Directions

Add all the ingredients except cucumber in a bowl and mix until well combined.

With a teaspoon, scoop out the center of each cucumber slice slightly.

Place the salmon mixture over each cucumber slice.

Serve immediately.

Zucchini Sticks

Total time: 40 minutes

Ingredients

2 large zucchinis, cut into 3-inch sticks lengthwise

Salt, as required

2 organic eggs

½ cup Parmesan cheese, grated

½ cup almonds, finely ground

½ teaspoon Italian herb seasoning

Directions

In a large colander, place the zucchini sticks and sprinkle with salt.

Set aside for about 1 hour to drain.

Preheat the oven to 425 degrees F. Line a baking sheet with parchment paper.

With your hands, squeeze the zucchini sticks to remove the excess liquid.

With a paper towel, pat dry the zucchini sticks.

Crack the eggs in a shallow bowl and beat them well.

Place the remaining ingredients in another bowl and mix until well combined.

Dip each zucchini sticks into the beaten eggs and then, evenly coat with the cheese mixture.

Arrange the zucchini sticks onto prepared baking sheet in a single layer.

Bake for 25 minutes, flipping once halfway through.

Remove from oven and transfer the zucchini sticks onto a platter.

Set aside to cool slightly.

Serve warm.

Broccoli Tots

Total time: 40 minutes

Ingredients

1 (16-ounces) package frozen chopped broccoli

3 large organic eggs

½ teaspoon dried oregano

½ teaspoon garlic powder

1/8 teaspoon cayenne pepper

1/8 teaspoon red pepper flakes, crushed

Salt and ground black pepper, as required

1 cup sharp cheddar cheese, grated

1 cup almond flour

Directions

Preheat the oven to 400 degrees F. Line two baking sheets with lightly greased parchment paper.

Place the broccoli into a microwave-safe bowl and microwave, covered for about 5 minutes, stirring once halfway through.

Drain the broccoli well.

Place the eggs, oregano, garlic powder, cayenne pepper, red pepper flakes, salt and black pepper in a large bowl and beat until well combined.

Add the cooked broccoli, cheddar cheese and almond flour and mix until well combined.

With slightly wet hands, make 24 equal-sized patties from the mixture.

Arrange the patties onto prepared baking sheets in a single layer about 2-inch apart.

Lightly, spray each patty with the cooking spray.

Bake for about 15 minutes per side or until golden brown from both sides.

Remove from oven and transfer the broccoli patties onto a platter.

Set aside to cool slightly.

Serve warm.

Cheesy Tomato Slices

Total time: 20 minutes

Ingredients

½ cup mayonnaise

½ cup ricotta cheese, shredded

½ cup part-skim mozzarella cheese, shredded

½ cup Parmesan and Romano cheese blend, grated

1 teaspoon garlic, minced

1 tablespoon dried oregano, crushed

Salt, as required

4 large tomatoes, cut each one in 5 slices

Directions

Preheat the broiler of oven on high. Arrange a rack about 3-inch from the heating element.

Place the mayonnaise, cheeses, garlic, oregano and salt in a bowl and mix until well combined and smooth.

Spread the cheese mixture evenly over each tomato slice.

Arrange the tomato slices onto broiler pan in a single layer.

Broil for about 3-5 minutes or until top becomes golden brown.

Remove from oven and transfer the tomato slices onto a platter.

Set aside to cool slightly.

Serve warm.

Stuffed Tomatoes

Total time: 30 minutes

Ingredients

24 cherry tomatoes

3 ounces cream cheese, softened

2 tablespoons mayonnaise

¼ cup cucumber, peeled and finely chopped

1 tablespoon scallion, finely chopped

2 teaspoons fresh dill, minced

Directions

Carefully, cut a thin slice from the top of each cherry tomato.

With the tip of a knife, carefully remove the pulp of each cherry tomato and discard it.

Arrange the tomatoes onto paper towels to drain, cut side down.

Place the cream cheese and mayonnaise in a bowl and beat until smooth.

Add the cucumber, scallion, and dill and stir to combine.

With a spoon, place the cheese mixture into each tomato.

Arrange the tomatoes onto a platter and refrigerate to chill slightly before serving.

Serve.

Bacon Wrapped Asparagus

Total time: 30 minutes

Ingredients

10 bacon slices, halved crosswise

6 ounces cream cheese, softened

1 (8-ounces) package frozen asparagus spears, thawed

Directions

Preheat the oven to 400 degrees F. Line two baking sheet with parchment paper.

Arrange the bacon slices onto a smooth surface.

Spread the cream cheese onto each bacon slice half.

Wrap each asparagus spear with 1 bacon slice half.

Arrange the wrapped asparagus onto prepared baking sheets in a single layer.

Bake for about 15 minutes.

Remove from the oven and serve warm.

Mini Mushroom Pizzas

Total time: 40 minutes

Ingredients

4 large Portobello mushrooms, stems removed

½ cup sugar-free marinara sauce

½ cup mozzarella cheese, shredded

1 gluten-free chorizo link, cut into thin slices

Directions

Preheat the oven to 375 degrees F. Line a large baking sheet with a lightly greased parchment paper.

With a spoon, scrape out the dark gills from mushrooms and discard the gills.

Arrange the mushrooms onto prepared baking sheet, stem side up.

Top each mushroom with the marinara sauce, followed by mozzarella and chorizo slices.

Bake for about 20-25 minutes or until the cheese is bubbly.

Remove from the oven and serve immediately.

Jalapeño Poppers

Total time: 40 minutes

Ingredients

10 ounces gluten-free pork sausage

½ cup cheddar cheese, shredded

24 fresh jalapeño peppers, stemmed and cut a slit along one side

12 bacon slices, halved lengthwise

Directions

Heat a medium nonstick skillet over medium heat and cook the sausage for about 8-10 minutes, breaking the links with spoon.

Drain the grease from skillet completely.

Remove the skillet from heat and let it cool completely.

Preheat the grill to medium heat. Grease the grill grate.

Add the cheddar cheese into cooled sausage and stir to combine.

Stuff each jalapeño pepper with the sausage mixture.

Wrap each jalapeño pepper with 1 halved bacon slice.

With a toothpick, secure each jalapeño pepper.

Place the jalapeño peppers onto grill and cook for about 15 minutes, flipping occasionally.

Remove from grill and transfer the jalapeño poppers onto a platter.

Set aside to cool slightly.

Serve warm.

Mozzarella Sticks

Total time: 16 minutes

Ingredients

8 bacon slices

8 mozzarella cheese sticks, frozen overnight

1 cup olive oil

Directions

Wrap a bacon slice around each cheese stick and secure with a toothpick.

In a cast iron skillet, heat the oil over medium heat and fry the mozzarella sticks in 2 batches for about 2-3 minutes or until golden brown from all sides.

With a slotted spoon, transfer the mozzarella sticks onto a paper towel-lined plate to drain.

Set aside to cool slightly.

Serve warm.

Cheese Balls

Total time: 27 minutes

Ingredients

2 organic eggs

½ cup cheddar cheese, shredded

¼ cup Parmesan cheese, shredded

¼ cup mozzarella cheese, shredded

½ cup almond flour

½ teaspoon organic baking powder

Ground black pepper, as required

Directions

Preheat the oven to 400 degrees F. Line a medium baking sheet with parchment paper.

Add the eggs into a large bowl and beat lightly.

Now, place the remaining ingredients and mix until well combined.

Make 8 equal-sized balls from the mixture.

Arrange the balls onto prepared baking sheet in a single layer.

Bake for about 10-12 minutes or until golden brown.

Remove from oven and transfer the cheese balls onto a platter.

Set aside to cool slightly.

Serve warm.

Parmesan Chicken Wings

Total time: 1 hour 15 minutes

Ingredients

3 pounds grass-fed chicken wings

1½ tablespoons organic baking powder

Salt and ground black pepper, as required

¼ cup salted butter

4 garlic cloves, minced

2 teaspoons dried parsley

Pinch of red pepper flakes

½ cup Parmesan cheese, grated

2 tablespoons fresh rosemary, chopped

Directions

Preheat the oven to 250 degrees F. Arrange an oven rack in the lower third of oven

Arrange a greased wire rack over a foil lined baking sheet.

Place the wings, baking powder, salt and black pepper in a ziplock bag.

Seal the bag and shake to coat well.

Now, arrange the wings onto prepared baking rack in a single layer.

Bake for about 30 minutes.

Now, increase the temperature of oven to 425 degrees F.

Then, arrange the baking sheet into the upper third of oven.

Bake for about 20-30 minutes or until crispy.

Meanwhile, place the butter, garlic, parsley and red pepper flakes in a bowl and mix well.

Remove from oven and transfer the wings into a large bowl.

Top the wings with butter mixture and parmesan and toss to coat well.

Garnish with fresh rosemary and serve immediately.

Buffalo Chicken Bites

Total time: 28 minutes

Ingredients

1 pound grass-fed ground chicken

1/3 cup almond flour

¼ cup Parmesan cheese, shredded

1 organic egg

1 tablespoon fresh chives, minced

1 garlic clove, minced

¼ teaspoon onion powder

½ cup hot sauce

2 tablespoons butter, melted

½ cup sugar-free ranch dressing

Directions

Preheat the oven to 500 degrees F. Grease one large baking sheet.

Place the ground chicken, almond flour, Parmesan cheese, egg, chives, garlic, and onion powder in a bowl and with your hands, mix until well combined.

Make 12 equal-sized balls from the mixture.

In the prepared baking sheet, arrange the meatballs in a single layer.

Bake for about 13 minutes or until the meatballs are done completely.

Meanwhile, add the hot sauce and butter in a large bowl and beat until well combined.

Remove the baking sheet of meatballs from oven and set aside for about 2-3 minutes.

Add meatballs into the bowl of hot sauce mixture and gently, toss to coat.

Transfer the meatballs onto a platter and drizzle with ranch dressing.

Serve immediately.

Mini Salmon Bites

Total time: 25 minutes

Ingredients

8 ounces cream cheese, softened

4 ounces smoked salmon, chopped

2 medium scallions, thinly sliced

Bagel seasoning, as required

Directions

In a bowl, add the cream cheese and beat until fluffy.

Add the smoked salmon, and scallions and beat until well combined.

Make bite-sized balls from the mixture and lightly coat with the bagel seasoning.

Arrange the balls onto 2 parchment-lined baking sheets and refrigerate for about 2-3 hours before serving.

Enjoy!

Tilapia Strips

Total time: 35 minutes

Ingredients

1 pound tilapia fillets, cut into strips

1 cup almond flour

Salt and ground black pepper, as required

2 large organic eggs, beaten

1½ cups Parmesan cheese, shredded

Directions

Preheat the oven to 450 degrees F. Line one baking sheet with parchment paper.

Place the almond flour, salt, and black pepper in a shallow bowl and mix until well combined.

Place the eggs and a splash of water in a second bowl and beat well.

Add the Parmesan cheese in a third bowl.

Coat the tilapia strips with flour mixture, then dip into the beaten eggs and finally, coat with cheese.

Arrange the tilapia strips onto prepared baking sheet in a single layer.

Bake for about 18-20 minutes or until done completely.

Remove from oven and transfer the tilapia strips onto a platter.

Set aside to cool slightly.

Serve warm.

Coconut Shrimp

Total time: 40 minutes

Ingredients

2 tablespoons coconut flour

Salt and ground black pepper, as required

2 large organic egg whites

1 cup unsweetened coconut flakes

1 pound shrimp, peeled and deveined

Directions

Preheat the oven to 400 degrees F. Grease one large baking sheet.

Place the coconut flour, salt and black pepper in a shallow bowl and mix until well combined.

Place the egg whites in a second bowl and beat until soft peaks form.

Add the coconut flakes in a third bowl.

Coat the shrimp with flour, then dip into the beaten egg whites and finally, coat with coconut flakes.

Arrange the shrimp onto prepared baking sheet in a single layer.

Bake for about 15 minutes.

Remove from oven and flip the shrimp.

Now, set the oven to broiler.

Broil the shrimp for about 3-5 minutes

Remove from oven and transfer the shrimp onto a platter.

Set aside to cool slightly.

Serve warm.

Bacon Wrapped Scallops

Total time: 35 minutes

Ingredients

18 sea scallops, side muscles removed

9 bacon slices, cut in half crosswise

2 tablespoons olive oil

Salt and ground black pepper, as required

Directions

Preheat the oven to 425 degrees F. Line a baking sheet with parchment paper.

Wrap each scallop with 1 bacon slice half and secure with toothpicks.

Drizzle the scallops evenly with oil and then, season with salt and black pepper.

Arrange scallops onto the prepared baking sheet in a single layer.

Bake for about 12-15 minutes or until scallop is tender and opaque.

Remove from the oven and serve immediately.

Chapter 12: Dinner Recipes

Shrimp & Bacon Chowder

Total time: 30 minutes

Ingredients

- ☐ Bacon – 6 slices, chopped
- ☐ Medium turnip – 1, cut into ½ cubes
- ☐ Chopped onion – ½ cup
- ☐ Garlic – 2 cloves, minced
- ☐ Chicken broth – 2 cups
- ☐ Heavy whipping cream – 1 cup
- ☐ Shrimp – 1 pound, peeled and deveined
- ☐ Cajun seasoning – ½ tsp.
- ☐ Salt and pepper
- ☐ Chopped parsley for garnish

Directions

Cook bacon in a Dutch oven until crisp. Remove and drain on paper towels. Reserve the bacon fat in the pan.

Add the onion and turnip and sauté for 5 minutes, or until onion is tender. Add garlic and cook until fragrant.

Pour in chicken broth and simmer for 10 minutes.

Add shrimp and cream and simmer for another 3 minutes, or until shrimp is cooked through.

Add Cajun seasoning and season with salt and pepper.

Garnish with chopped parsley and bacon and serve.

Creamy Salmon

Total time: 30 minutes

Ingredients

- ☐ Olive oil – 2 Tbsp.

- ☐ Salmon fillets – 3 (6-ounce)

- ☐ Garlic – 2 cloves, minced

- ☐ Heavy whipping cream – 1 cup

- ☐ Cream cheese – 1 ounce

- ☐ Capers – 2 Tbsp.

- ☐ Lemon juice – 1 Tbsp.

- ☐ Fresh dill – 2 tsp.

- ☐ Grated Parmesan cheese – 2 Tbsp.

Directions

Heat oil in a skillet. Add the salmon and search each side for 5 minutes.

Once cooked, remove and set aside.

Add the minced garlic to the pan and sauté until fragrant.

Add the capers, lemon juice, cream cheese, and heavy cream to the pan.

Bring to a light simmer. Stir frequently.

Once the sauce starts to thicken, add the salmon back in the pan. Coat the salmon with the sauce and just reheat the fish.

Garnish with Parmesan cheese and fresh dill and serve.

Orange Chicken

Total time: 25 minutes

Ingredients (*chicken*)

☐ Chicken thighs – 2 pounds, skinless, boneless, and cut into pieces

☐ Salt and ground black pepper to taste

☐ Coconut oil – 3 Tbsp.

☐ Coconut flour – ¼ cup

Ingredients (sauce)

☐ Fish sauce – 2 Tbsp.

☐ Lemon zest – 1 ½ tsp.

☐ Fresh ginger - 1 Tbsp. grated

- [ ] Orange juice – ¼ cup, no sugar added

- [ ] Stevia – 2 tsp.

- [ ] Sesame seeds – ¼ tsp.

- [ ] Scallions – 2 Tbsp. chopped

- [ ] Coriander – ½ tsp.

- [ ] Water – 1 cup

- [ ] Red pepper flakes – ¼ tsp.

- [ ] Liquid aminos – 2 Tbsp.

Directions

In a bowl, mix coconut flour, salt, pepper, and stir.

Add chicken pieces and toss to coat well.

Heat a pan with oil. Add chicken, and cook until golden brown on both sides. Transfer to a bowl.

In a blender, mix orange juice with ginger, fish sauce, liquid aminos, stevia, lemon zest, water, coriander, and blend well.

Pour into a pan and heat over medium heat.

Add chicken, stir, and cook for 2 minutes.

Add sesame seeds, scallions, and pepper flakes. Stir-fry for 2 minutes. Remove from heat.

Serve.

Duck with Sauce

Total time: 30 minutes

Ingredients

- ☐ Duck breasts – 2

- ☐ Salt – 1 tsp.

- ☐ Pepper – ½ tsp.

- ☐ Chinese 5 spice – 1.5 tsp.

Ingredients (sauce)

- ☐ Chicken stock – 1 cup

- ☐ Xylitol – 2 Tbsp.

- ☐ Tamari – 4 Tbsp.

- ☐ Chinese 5 spice – ½ tsp.

- ☐ Cinnamon – ½ tsp.

- ☐ Apple cider vinegar – 2 tsp.

- ☐ Peel of one orange

Directions

Preheat the oven to 400F.

Combine all the sauce ingredients in a small saucepan.

Simmer the sauce for 20 to 25 minutes on low heat while you prepare the duck. Whisk occasionally.

To prepare the duck, combine salt, pepper, and 5 spice.

Score the duck skin (similar to crisscross pattern).

Rub the duck breast well with the spice mixture.

Heat a pan and place the duck breasts, skin side down.

Cook for 5 minutes, then turn and cook for 2 minutes more. Drain off the fat.

Cook the duck in the oven for 8 to 10 minutes.

Remove from the oven. Cover with a foil and rest. Discard the orange peel.

Serve with a salad.

Pan-Seared Steak

Total time: 15 minutes

Ingredients

☐   Steak (filet, sirloin strip, ribeye) – 6 oz. (about 1 inch thick)

☐   Salted butter – 2 Tbsp.

☐   Sliced shiitake mushrooms – ½ cup

☐   Kosher salt and pepper to taste

Directions

Heat a cast-iron pan on medium heat for 1 minute.

Season the steak with salt and pepper and add to the hot pan.

Cook 3 to 4 minutes for medium-rare.

Remove the steak to a plate.

Add butter and mushrooms to the pan.

Cook until the mushrooms are golden brown, about 3 to 4 minutes. Remove from the heat.

Season the mushroom with salt and pepper if needed.

Add the steak back to the pan and baste in the butter.

Allow to rest in the warm butter for a couple of minutes.

Slice and serve.

Slow Cooked Beef Pot Roast

Total time: 7 hours 30 minutes

Ingredients:

- 2 pounds beef pot roast, cut

- 2 tablespoon beef tallow

- ½ teaspoon black pepper

- ½ teaspoon dried oregano

- 1 tablespoon dried thyme

- 1 teaspoon salt

- 1 whole bay leaf

- 1 medium onion, sliced

- 3 cups water

Directions:

In a bowl, mix together thyme, black pepper, oregano and salt.

Rub the mixture all over the pot roast cut.

Heat a skillet and melt the beef tallow. Place the marinated pot roast and sear all sides.

Meanwhile, put remaining ingredients in slow cooker.

Add the seared pot roast and cook for 7 hours.

Let it cool. Evenly divide into suggested servings and place in meal prep containers.

Stuffed Instant Pot Chicken Breasts

Total time: 55 minutes

Ingredients:

- 1-piece ham, halved

- 16 strips bacon

- 2 cups water

- 2 strips of skinless chicken breasts

- 4 slices mozzarella cheese

- 6 asparagus spears, trimmed

- 1 tablespoon salt

Directions:

Butterfly the chicken breasts by placing them on a chopping board and slicing the breasts horizontally. Place a plastic wrap over the chicken breasts and use a meat mallet to pound the breasts flatter.

In a mixing bowl, mix 1 tablespoon of salt and water. Soak the butterflied chicken breasts in the brine for 30 minutes. Pat dry the chicken breasts after marinating in the brine.

Lay the chicken breasts on a flat surface and place 1 halved of ham, 2 slices of mozzarella cheese, and 3 spears of asparagus on the center.

Roll up the chicken breasts and secure the edges with toothpick. Roll the bacon around the rolled chicken breasts and secure with more toothpicks.

Place a steamer rack or trivet in the Instant Pot and pour 1 cup of cold water. Place the chicken roll ups on the steamer rack.

Close the lid and select manual. Cook on high pressure for 7 minutes and do natural release. Take the roll ups out from the Instant Pot. Place the chicken roll ups in the fridge for an hour. Remove the toothpicks.

Drain out the pot from the water and remove the steamer rack.

Set the sauté setting on the Instant Pot and add the chicken roll ups. Sauté until the bacon renders its own oil.

Let it cool. Evenly divide into suggested servings and place in meal prep containers.

Slow Cooker Balsamic Roast Beef

Total time: 8 hours 15 minutes

Ingredients:

- 1 ¾ pound boneless round roast

- 1 cup beef broth

- 1 tablespoon Stevia

- 1 tablespoon soy sauce

- 1 tablespoon Worcestershire sauce

- 4 cloves chopped garlic

- ¼ teaspoon red pepper flakes

Directions:

Place the roast beef in the slow cooker.

In a mixing bowl, mix all other ingredients and pour over the roast.

Let it sit in the slow cooker for six to eight hours.

Once cooked, remove from the slow cooker and break the meat apart.

Let it cool. Evenly divide into suggested servings and place in meal prep containers.

Buffalo Turkey Balls

Total time: 50 minutes

Ingredients:

- 2 eggs

- 1-lb ground turkey

- ½ cup hot sauce

- ½ stick unsalted butter

- ¼ cup almond flour

- 3 tablespoon blue cheese, crumbled

- 2-oz whipped cream cheese

Directions:

Preheat the oven at 350 degrees Fahrenheit.

Mix the turkey meat, cream cheese, egg, blue cheese and almond flour in a mixing bowl. Mix well and evenly divide into 20 small meat balls.

Place the meat balls on a greased baking spray.

Bake for 15 minutes.

While the meatball is baking, make the sauce by mixing the butter and hot sauce in a sauce pan.

Remove the turkey balls from the oven and dip them in the hot sauce.

Place the turkey balls in the oven and re-bake for another 15 minutes.

Let it cool. Evenly divide into suggested servings and place in meal prep containers.

Stuffed Enchilada Peppers

Ingredients:

- 6 red or yellow peppers

- ½ cup green chilies

- 1 can fat-free plain Greek yogurt

- 1 cup fresh spinach, chopped

- 1 cup cauliflower rice

- 1-lb shredded cooked turkey or chicken breast

- 1 package shredded cheese

Directions:

Lightly grease a cookie sheet with cooking spray and preheat oven to 375ºF.

Cut the tops of each pepper and remove the seeds. Set aside.

In a mixing bowl, mix together spinach, cheese, meat, cauliflower rice, and yogurt.

Fill the hollowed peppers with 2/3 of the meat mixture. Put the tops of the pepper back on.

Place the peppers on prepared cookie sheet and pop in the oven. Bake for 25 minutes.

Let it cool. Evenly divide into suggested servings and place in meal prep containers.

Keto Chicken Adobo

Total time: 40 minutes

Ingredients:

- 8 skinless chicken drumsticks

- ¼ cup coconut aminos

- ½ teaspoon cracked black pepper

- 1 tablespoon olive oil

- 1 red onion, chopped

- ¼ cup vinegar

- 2 bay leaves

- ½ cup water

- 8 garlic cloves, crushed

Directions:

Place a medium pot on medium high heat and heat oil.

Once hot, sauté garlic for a minute.

Add onion and sauté until wilted, around 5 minutes.

Stir in bay leaves and cracked pepper.

Add chicken and sauté for 8 minutes.

Add coconut aminos and vinegar. Continue cooking until liquid is halved.

Add water, bring to a simmer, cover, and cook for 15 minutes.

Let it cool. Evenly divide into suggested servings and place in meal prep containers.

Basil Tomato Frittata

Total time: 25 minutes

Ingredients

5 eggs

1 tbsp olive oil

7 oz can artichokes

1 garlic clove, chopped

1 onion, chopped

1/2 cup cherry tomatoes

2 tbsp fresh basil, chopped

1/4 cup feta cheese, crumbled

1/4 tsp pepper

1/4 tsp salt

Directions:

Heat oil in a pan over medium heat.

Add garlic and onion and sauté for 4 minutes.

Add artichokes, basil, and tomatoes and cook for 4 minutes.

Beat eggs in a bowl and season with pepper and salt.

Pour egg mixture into the pan and cook for 5-7 minutes.

Serve and enjoy.

Chia Spinach Pancakes

Total time: 15 minutes

Ingredients

4 eggs

½ cup coconut flour

1 cup coconut milk

¼ cup chia seeds

1 cup spinach, chopped

1 tsp baking soda

½ tsp pepper

½ tsp salt

Directions:

Whisk eggs in a bowl until frothy.

Combine together all dry ingredients and add in egg mixture and whisk until smooth. Add spinach and stir well.

Greased pan with butter and heat over medium heat.

Pour 3-4 tablespoons of batter onto the pan and make pancake.

Cook pancake until lightly golden brown from both the sides.

Serve and enjoy.

Feta Kale Frittata

Total time: 2 hours 20 minutes

Ingredients

8 eggs, beaten

4 oz feta cheese, crumbled

6 oz bell pepper, roasted and diced

5 oz baby kale

1/4 cup green onion, sliced

2 tsp olive oil

Directions:

Heat olive oil in a pan over medium-high heat.

Add kale to the pan and sauté for 4-5 minutes or until softened.

Spray slow cooker with cooking spray.

Add cooked kale into the slow cooker.

Add green onion and bell pepper into the slow cooker.

Pour beaten eggs into the slow cooker and stir well to combine.

Sprinkle crumbled feta cheese.

Cook on low for 2 hours or until frittata is set.

Serve and enjoy.

Protein Muffins

Total time: 25 minutes

Ingredients

8 eggs

2 scoop vanilla protein powder

8 oz cream cheese

4 tbsp butter, melted

Directions:

In a large bowl, combine together cream cheese and melted butter.

Add eggs and protein powder and whisk until well combined.

Pour batter into the greased muffin pan.

Bake at 350 F for 25 minutes.

Serve and enjoy.

Healthy Waffles

Total time: 20 minutes

Ingredients

8 drops liquid stevia

1/2 tsp baking soda

1 tbsp chia seeds

1/4 cup water

2 tbsp sunflower seed butter

1 tsp cinnamon

1 avocado, peel, pitted and mashed

1 tsp vanilla

1 tbsp lemon juice

3 tbsp coconut flour

Directions:

Preheat the waffle iron.

In a small bowl, add water and chia seeds and soak for 5 minutes.

Mash together sunflower seed butter, lemon juice, vanilla, stevia, chia mixture, and avocado.

Mix together cinnamon, baking soda, and coconut flour.

Add wet ingredients to the dry ingredients and mix well.

Pour waffle mixture into the hot waffle iron and cook on each side for 3-5 minutes.

Serve and enjoy.

Cheese Zucchini Eggplant

Total time: 2 hours 10 minutes

Ingredients

1 eggplant, peeled and cut in 1-inch cubes

1 ½ cup spaghetti sauce

1 onion, sliced

1 medium zucchini, cut into 1-inch pieces

1/2 cup parmesan cheese, shredded

Directions:

Add all ingredients into the crock pot and stir well.

Cover and cook on high for 2 hours.

Stir well and serve.

Coconut Kale Muffins

Total time: 40 minutes

Ingredients

6 eggs

1/2 cup unsweetened coconut milk

1 cup kale, chopped

¼ tsp garlic powder

¼ tsp paprika

1/4 cup green onion, chopped

Pepper

Salt

Directions:

Preheat the oven to 350 F.

Add all ingredients into the bowl and whisk well.

Pour mixture into the greased muffin tray and bake in oven for 30 minutes.

Blueberry Muffins

Total time: 35 minutes

Ingredients

2 eggs

½ tsp vanilla

1/2 cup fresh blueberries

1 tsp baking powder

6 drops stevia

1 cup heavy cream

2 cups almond flour

1/4 cup butter, melted

Directions:

Preheat the oven to 350 F.

Add eggs to the mixing bowl and whisk until well mix.

Add remaining ingredients to the eggs and mix well to combine.

Pour batter into greased muffin tray and bake in oven for 25 minutes.

Serve and enjoy.

Coconut Bread

Total time: 45 minutes

Ingredients

6 eggs

1 tbsp baking powder

2 tbsp swerve

1/2 cup ground flaxseed

1/2 cup coconut flour

1/2 tsp cinnamon

1 tsp xanthan gum

1/3 cup unsweetened coconut milk

1/2 cup olive oil

1/2 tsp salt

Directions:

Preheat the oven to 375 F.

Add eggs, milk, and oil into the stand mixer and blend until combined.

Add remaining ingredients and blend until well mixed.

Pour batter in greased loaf pan.

Bake in oven for 40 minutes.

Slice and serve.

Pumpkin Muffins

Total time: 35 minutes

Ingredients

4 eggs

1/2 cup pumpkin puree

1 tsp pumpkin pie spice

1/2 cup almond flour

1 tbsp baking powder

1 tsp vanilla

1/3 cup coconut oil, melted

2/3 cup swerve

1/2 cup coconut flour

1/2 tsp sea salt

Directions:

Preheat the oven to 350 F.

In a large bowl, stir together coconut flour, pumpkin pie spice, baking powder, swerve, almond flour, and sea salt.

Stir in eggs, vanilla, coconut oil, and pumpkin puree until well combined.

Pour batter into the greased muffin tray and bake in oven for 25 minutes.

Serve and enjoy.

Broccoli Nuggets

Total time: 25 minutes

Ingredients

2 egg whites

2 cups broccoli florets

1/4 cup almond flour

1 cup cheddar cheese, shredded

1/8 tsp salt

Directions:

Preheat the oven to 350 F.

Add broccoli in bowl and mash using masher.

Add remaining ingredients to the broccoli and mix well.

Drop 20 scoops onto baking tray and press lightly down.

Bake in preheated oven for 20 minutes.

Serve and enjoy.

Cheesy Spinach Quiche

Total time: 7 hour 10 minutes

Ingredients

8 eggs

2 cups fresh spinach

1/2 cup feta cheese, crumbled

1/2 cup parmesan cheese, shredded

1/4 cup cheddar cheese, shredded

3 garlic cloves, minced

2 cups unsweetened almond milk

1/4 tsp salt

Directions:

In a large bowl, whisk together eggs and almond milk.

Add spinach, parmesan cheese, feta cheese, garlic, and salt and stir well to combine.

Spray crock potwith cooking spray.

Pour egg mixture into the crock pot.

Sprinkle shredded cheddar cheese over the top of egg mixture.

Cover and cook on low for 7 hours.

Vegetable Quiche

Total time: 40 minutes

Ingredients

8 eggs

1 onion, chopped

1 cup Parmesan cheese, grated

1 cup unsweetened coconut milk

1 cup tomatoes, chopped

1 cup zucchini, chopped

1 tbsp butter

1/2 tsp pepper

1 tsp salt

Directions:

Preheat the oven to 400 F.

Melt butter in a pan over medium heat then add onion and sauté until onion soften.

Add tomatoes and zucchini to pan and sauté for 4 minutes.

Beat eggs with cheese, milk, pepper and salt in a bowl.

Pour egg mixture over vegetables and bake in oven for 30 minutes.

Slices and serve.

Coconut Porridge

Total time: 15 minutes

Ingredients

1 cup unsweetened shredded coconut

1/4 tsp cinnamon

1 tsp vanilla

2 cups unsweetened coconut milk

1/4 cup psyllium husks

1/4 cup coconut flour

28 drops liquid stevia

1/4 tsp nutmeg

2 2/3 cups water

Directions:

Add coconut in pot and toast over medium-high heat.

Add water and coconut milk and stir well. Cover and bring to boil.

When it begins to boiling then remove from heat.

Add remaining ingredients and stir well.

Serve and enjoy.

Baked Eggplant Zucchini

Total time: 50 minutes

Ingredients

3 medium zucchini, sliced

1/4 cup parsley, chopped

1/4 cup basil, chopped

1 cup cherry tomatoes, halved

1 medium eggplant, sliced

1 tbsp olive oil

3 oz parmesan cheese, grated

3 garlic cloves, minced

1/4 tsp pepper

1/4 tsp salt

Directions:

Preheat the oven to 350 F.

In a bowl, add cherry tomatoes, eggplant, zucchini, olive oil, garlic, cheese, basil, pepper, and salt toss well until combined.

Transfer eggplant mixture into greased baking dish.

Bake in oven for 35 minutes.

Garnish withparsley and serve.

Cheese Broccoli Bread

Total time: 35 minutes

Ingredients

5 eggs, lightly beaten

2 tsp baking powder

4 tbsp coconut flour

1 cup broccoli florets, chopped

1 cup cheddar cheese, shredded

Directions:

Preheat the oven to 350 F.

Add all ingredients into the bowl and mix well.

Pour egg mixture into the prepared loaf pan and bake in oven for 30 minutes.

Slice and serve.

Shrimp Green Beans

Total time: 20 minutes

Ingredients

1 lb shrimp, peeled and deveined

1 ½ tbsp soy sauce

2 tbsp olive oil

1/2 lb green beans, trimmed

Salt

Directions:

Heat oil in a pan over medium-high heat.

Add beans to the pan and sauté for 5-6 minutes.

Remove pan from heat and set aside.

Add shrimp in the same pan and sauté for 2-3 minutes each side.

Return beans to the pan.

Add soy sauce and stir well and cook shrimp is completely cooked.

Season with salt. Serve.

Easy Asparagus Quiche

Total time: 70 minutes

Ingredients

14 asparagus spears, cut ends and halved

5 eggs, beaten

1 cup unsweetened almond milk

1 cup cheddar cheese, shredded

1/4 tsp salt

Directions:

Preheat the oven to 350 F.

In a bowl, beat together eggs, thyme, white pepper, almond milk, and salt.

Arrange asparagus in greased quiche dish then pour egg mixture over asparagus.

Sprinkle cheese on top and bake for 60 minutes.

Slices and serve.

Olive Cheese Omelet

Total time: 15 minutes

Ingredients

4 large eggs

2 oz cheese

12 olives, pitted

2 tbsp butter

2 tbsp olive oil

1 tsp herb de Provence

1/2 tsp salt

Directions:

Add all ingredients except butter in a bowl whisk well until frothy.

Melt butter in a pan over medium heat.

Pour egg mixture onto hot pan and spread evenly.

Cover and cook for 3 minutes.

Turn omelet to other side and cook for 2 minutes more.

Serve and enjoy.

Cheese Almond Pancakes

Total time: 20 minutes

Ingredients

4 eggs

1/4 tsp cinnamon

1/2 cup cream cheese

1/2 cup almond flour

1 tbsp butter, melted

Directions:

Add all ingredients into the blender and blend until combined.

Melt butter in a pan over medium heat.

Pour 3 tablespoons of batter per pancake and cook for 2 minutes on each side.

Serve and enjoy.

Cauliflower Frittata

Total time: 15 minutes

Ingredients

1 egg

1/2 tbsp onion, diced

¼ cup cauliflower rice

1 tbsp olive oil

1/4 tsp turmeric

Pepper

Salt

Directions:

Add all ingredients except oil into the bowl and mix well to combine.

Heat oil in a pan over medium heat.

Pour the mixture into the hot oil pan and cook for 3-4 minutes or until lightly golden brown.

Serve and enjoy.

Chapter 13 : Dessert Recipes

Keto Mocha Brownies

Total time: 55 minutes

Ingredients

For the base:

6 eggs; separated

3 tbsp butter; unsalted

2 tsp baking powder

1 ½ cup swerve

1 ½ cups of almond flour

1/4 tsp salt

For the topping:

1 ½ cup swerve or stevia crystal

2 butter sticks; unsalted

1/4 cup black coffee; unsweetened

5 egg yolks

Directions:

Place egg whites in a large mixing bowl and beat on medium speed until light and fluffy. Add swerve, almond glour, melted butter, baking powder, and salt.

Beat well on medium-high speed until completely incporporated

Line a small cake pan with some parchment paper and add the batter. Tightly wrap with aluminum foil and set aside

Plug in the instant pot and position a trivet at the bottom of the inner pot. Pour in some water and add the cake pan

Securely seal the lid and set the steam release handle to the *Sealing* position. Press the *Manual* button and set the timer for 15 minutes on high pressure

When done; perform a quick pressure release and open the lid. Remove the pan from the pot and set aside to cool

Now place a steam basket in the stainless steel insert and pour in some more water, Set aside

In a large mixing bowl, combine together the filling ingredients. With a whisking attachment on, beat well on medium-high speed for 2 - 3 minutes

Pour the mixture into an oven-safe bowl and wrap with aluminum foil. Place the bowl in the steam basket and seal the lid.

Set the steam release handle and cook for 4 minutes on the *Manual* mode

When you hear the cooker's end signal, perform a quick pressure release and open the lid. Remove the bowl from the pot and chill for a while

Pour the mixture over the crust and cool to a room temperature. Refrigerate for at least an hour before serving.

Keto Raspberry Cheesecake

Total time: 2 hours 30 minutes

Ingredients

1 cup almond flour

1/4 cup almond butter

5 eggs

3 tsp stevia powder

1/4 cup sunflower seeds

1/4 tsp salt

For the filling:

4 tbsp stevia powder

3 cups cream cheese

1 tsp raspberry extract

1/2 cup heavy cream

1 tsp agar powder

Directions:

Line a fitting springform pan with some parchment paper and grease the walls with some cooking spray, Set aside

In a large mixing bowl, combine almond flour, sunflower seeds, stevia, and salt. Using a spatula, mix until well incorporated, Set aside

In a separate bowl, combine eggs and butter. With a whisking attachment on, beat with a hand mixer for 3 - 4 minutes.

Now; pour egg mixture into dry ingredients. With a paddle attachment on, beat until combined.

Transfer the dough mixture to the springform pan and spread evenly, Set aside

In a large mixing bowl, combine all filing ingredients and beat for 3 minutes with a hand mixer. Pour the filling over the crust

Plug in the instant pot and pour 1 cup of water in the stainless steel insert. Set the trivet on the bottom. Place the springform pan on the top and seal the lid. Adjust the steam release handle and press the *Slow Cook* button. Set the timer for 2 hours and cook on *Low* pressure

When you hear the cooker's end signal, perform a quick pressure release and open the pot. Transfer the pan to a wire rack and let it chill for at least an hour. Refrigerate for 30 minutes before serving.

Optionally, top with some fresh raspberries.

Choco Cinnamon Cake

Total time: 50 minutes

Ingredients

1 cup coconut flour

1/2 cup granulated stevia

1/2 cup almonds; minced

4 tbsp almond butter

1/2 cup cream cheese

1 tbsp unsweetened cocoa powder

2 large eggs

1/4 tsp apple pie spice

1/4 tsp cinnamon; ground

1/4 tsp salt

Directions:

Combine coconut flour, almonds, granulated stevia, salt, cinnamon, and apple pie spice in a large mixing bowl. Using a spatula, mix until combined

Gradually, add eggs, butter, and cream cheese. Beat with a hand mixer until well incorporated.

Plug in your instant pot and pour 1 cup of water in the stainless steel insert. Set the trivet on the bottom.

Line a fitting springform pan with some parchment paper and grease the walls with some cooking spray. Pour in the mixture and cover the top with some aluminum foil

Set the pan on top of the trivet and close the lid. Adjust the steam release handle and press the *Manual* button. Set the timer for 35 minutes on *High* pressure

When you hear the cooker's end signal, perform a quick pressure release and open the pot. Using oven mitts, remove the pan to a wire rack and let it cool completely

Sprinkle with cocoa and enjoy!

Delicious Raspberry Muffins with Chocolate Topping

Total time: 50 minutes

Ingredients

1 cup fresh raspberries

1/4 cup coconut butter; melted

1 cup almond flour

1/4 cup granulated stevia

2 large eggs

1 tsp vanilla extract

1/4 cup whole milk

1 tsp baking powder

1/4 tsp salt

For the topping:

1/4 tsp cinnamon; ground

1/4 cup dark chocolate chips; melted

1/4 cup butter

Directions:

In a large mixing bowl, combine almond flour, stevia, baking powder, and salt. Mix until combined and set aside

In a separate bowl, combine eggs, milk, and vanilla extract. Beat with a hand mixer until fluffy

Now; add the wet ingredients to the bowl with dry ingredients. Mix until you get a thick batter. Add raspberries and stir with a spatula

Pour the mixture in silicone muffin molds and set aside

Plug in the instant pot and pour 1 cup of water in the stainless steel insert. Set the trivet on the bottom and place molds on top.

Close the lid and adjust the steam release handle. Press the *Manual* button and set the timer for 30 minutes. Cook on *High* pressure

Meanwhile; combine all topping ingredients in a mixing bowl. Beat with a mixer until all well combined and creamy, Set aside

When you hear the cooker's end signal, perform a quick pressure release and open the pot.

Carefully transfer the muffins to a wire rack and let it cool completely

Using a pipping bag, swirl the mixture over each muffin. Refrigerate for 15 minutes before serving.

Amazing Keto Almond Coffee Cups

Total time: 50 minutes

Ingredients

For the crust:

1 cup almonds; minced

2 large eggs

1/2 cup shredded coconut

1 tbsp butter; softened

1/2 tsp vanilla extract

For the filling:

2 tsp stevia powder

1 tsp xanthan gum

1 cup heavy whipping cream

1 tsp instant black coffee; unsweetened

Directions:

First, prepare the topping. Plug in the instant pot and combine all filling ingredients in the stainless steel insert. Press the *Saute* button and gently stir. Cook for 2 - 3 minutes without boiling. Turn off the pot and transfer all to a large bowl. Refrigerate for 30 minutes. Clean the pot and set aside

Now; combine almonds and coconut in a large bowl. Mix with a spatula and add eggs. Using a hand mixer, beat until well combined. Add butter and vanilla extract. Beat again ntil well combined

Divide the mixture evenly between silicone muffin molds. Press with your fingers to form cups.

Pour 1 cup of water in the stainless steel insert and set the trivet on the bottom. Place the silicone molds on top and close the lid. Adjust the steam release handle and press the *Manual* button. Set the timer for 30 minutes and cook on *High* pressure

When done; perform a quick release of the pressure and open the pot. Transfer to a wire rack to cool completely. Spoon the filling onto each crust and refrigerate for 1 hour before serving.

Optionally, top with some fresh raspberries.

Keto Cherry Mousse

Total time: 20 minutes

Ingredients

1 ½ cup whipping cream

1/4 cup erythritol

5 large egg yolks; beaten

1/2 cup whole milk

1/2 cup coconut cream

1 tbsp pecans; minced

2 tsp cherry extract

1/2 tsp salt

Directions:

Combine whipping cream, egg yolks, erytthritol, milk, salt, and coconut cream in a medium-sized saucepan over a medium-high heat. Stir well and heat up without boiling. Remove from the heat and pour the mixture into oven-safe ramekins. Sprinkle with minced pecans and wrap each ramekin with aluminum foil, Set aside

Plug in your instant pot and pour 1 cup of water in the stainless steel insert. Set the trivet on the bottom and place the ramekins on top

Securely lock the lid and adjust the steam release handle by moving the valve to the *Sealing* position. Set the timer for 7 minutes on *Manual* mode

When you hear the cooker's end signal, perform a quick pressure release and open the pot. Transfer the ramekins to a wire rack and let it cool completely

Refrigerate for at least an hour before serving.

Chocolate Chip Pudding

Total time: 10 minutes

Ingredients

1 cup unsweetened almond milk

2 tbsp chocolate chips; sugar-free

1 tbsp agar powder

1 ¼ cup whipping cream

1/2 cup coconut cream

1/4 cup swerve

1/4 cup almonds; finely chopped.

2 tbsp cocoa powder; unsweetened

1 tsp vanilla extract

Directions:

Plug in the instant pot and pour in the milk. Press the *Saute* button and heat up. Add swerve, cocoa powder, coconut cream, and vanilla extract.

Bring it to a boil, stirring constantly, and then add agar powder. Continue to cook for 1 - 2 minutes.

Press the *Cancel'* button and stir in finely chopped almonds

Transfer the mixture to a large mixing bowl and pour in the whipping cream. Beat well on high speed for 2 - 3 minutes.

Finally, divide the mixture between serving bowls and cool completely before serving.

Tasty Crumbled Lemon Muffin Parfait

Preparation Time: 40 Minutes

Servings: 6

Ingredients:

1/4 cup almond flour

4 tbsp unsweetened raw cocoa

1/2 tsp baking powder

3 tbsp granulated stevia

1 tsp vanilla extract

2 large eggs

1/4 cup almond butter

For the creamy filling:

1 tsp lemon extract

1 tsp stevia powder

1 cup cream cheese

1/4 cup whipping cream

Directions:

In a large mixing bowl, combine almond flour, stevia, cocoa, and baking powder. Stir well and set aside

In a separate bowl, combine eggs, butter, and vanilla extract. Beat with a hand mixer until well combined. Now; add this mixture to the dry ingredients and mix well. Divide the mixture evenly between muffin molds and set aside

Plug in the instant pot and pour 1 cup of water in the stainless steel insert. Set the trivet on the bottom and place the molds on top. Close the lid and adjust the steam release handle. Press the *Manual* button and set the timer for 20 minutes on *High* pressure

Meanwhile, combine all filling ingredients in a large bowl. Beat with a hand mixer until smooth and creamy, Set aside

When you hear the cooker's end signal, perform a quick pressure release and open the pot. Transfer the molds to a wire rack and let it cool completely

Crumble the muffins into small pieces. Make a 1-inch thick layer with a muffin crumbles and top with 1-inch thick creamy filling. Repeat the process with the remaining mixture. Optionally, sprinkle the top with lemon zest.

Refrigerate for 1 hour before serving.

Sweet Potato & Cinnamon Patties

Total time: 30 minutes

Ingredients

1 small sweet potato; cubed

1 tbsp psyllium husk powder

1/2 cup Mascarpone

1/2 cup almond flour

3 tbsp granulated stevia

1/4 cup flaxseed meal

3 tbsp coconut oil; softened

1/2 tsp cinnamon powder

1 tsp vanilla extract

Directions:

Plug in the instant pot and add potatoes. Pour in enough water to cover and seal the lid. Set the steam release handle and cook for 3 minutes on the *Manual* mode

When done; perform a quick pressure release and open the lid

Remove potatoes from the pot and drain. Cool for a while and transfer to a food processor along with the remaining ingredients. Process until smooth.

Now press the *Saute* button and grease the inner pot with some oil. Add about 1/4 cup of the potato mixture and cook for 3 - 4 minutes on one side

Gently turn over and continue to cook for another 2 minutes.

Repeat the process with the remaining mixture

Optionally, sprinkle with some granulated stevia before serving.

Keto Coconut Bars

Total time: 25 minutes

Ingredients

2 cups shredded coconut

1 tbsp chia seeds

1/4 cup flaxseed meal

1/2 cup coconut oil

1 tbsp sesame seeds

1/4 cup almonds; finely chopped.

2 tbsp almond butter

3 large eggs

2 tbsp granulated stevia

1 tsp vanilla extract

1/4 tsp salt

Directions:

Combine the ingredients in a large bowl and mix until a lightly sticky mixture forms. Optionally, add some more stevia and set aside

Line a small baking pan with some parchment paper and lightly grease with some coconut oil. Add the mixture and press well with the palms of your hands to flatten the surface as evenly as possible

Loosely cover with aluminum foil and set aside

Plug in the instant pot and set the trivet at the bottom of the inner pot. Pour in two cups of water and place the baking pan

Seal the lid and set the steam release handle to the *Sealing* position. Cook for 15 minutes on the *Manual* mode

When done; perform a quick pressure release and open the lid. Remove the pan and cool to a room temperature before slicing into bars.

Refrigerate for one hour before serving.

Chocolate Bounties

Total time: 25 minutes

Ingredients

1 cup shredded coconut

1/2 cup heavy whipping cream

2 tbsp unsweetened cocoa powder

4 tbsp butter

1 tbsp hazelnuts; minced

1 tsp vanilla extract

1 tsp stevia powder

1/4 tsp salt

For the coating:

1 tsp lemon zest; freshly grated

1 tbsp shredded coconut

1 cup dark chocolate; 80% cocoa

2 tbsp heavy cream

Directions:

Plug in your instant pot and add butter to the stainless steel insert. Press the *Saute* button and stir with a wooden spatula until melts.

Add heavy whipping cream, cocoa, vanilla extract, and stevia powder. Heat up without boiling. Stir constantly

Turn off the pot and transfer all to a large mixing bowl. Add shredded coconut, salt, and hazelnuts. Mix until well combined and set aside

Clean the stainless steel insert and pour in 1 cup of water. Set the trivet on the bottom.

Combine chocolate, heavy cream, and lemon zest in an oven-safe ramekin. Place the ramekin on the top of the trivet and close the lid. Adjust the steam release handle and press the *Manual* button. Cook for 2 minutes on *High* pressure

When done; perform a quick pressure release and open the pot

Coat the walls of your ice tray with some chocolate. Fill with coconut mixture and then top with the remaining chocolate. Sprinkle with cconut and set aside to cool completely

Refrigerate for 2 hours before serving.

Lemon Cake

Total time: 50 minutes

Ingredients

For the cake:

3 cups almond flour

3 tsp baking powder

2 tsp lemon extract

1/4 cup butter; softened

5 large eggs

3 tbsp stevia powder

1/4 cup coconut milk; full-fat

1 tbsp coconut cream

1/4 tsp salt

For the syrup:

1 tbsp lemon juice; freshly squeeze

1/4 cup granulated stevia

1/4 cup raspberries

1/4 cup blueberries

Directions:

In a large mixing bowl, combine together almond flour, stevia powder, baking powder, and salt.

Mix well and add eggs, one at the time, beating constantly

Now add coconut milk, coconut cream, butter, and lemon extract. Using a paddle attachment beat for 3 minutes on medium speed

Grease a small cake pan with some oil and line with parchment paper. Pour the mixture in it and tightly wrap with aluminum foil.

Plug in the instant pot and set the trivet at the bottom of the inner pot. Place the cake pan on top and pour in one cup of water.

Seal the lid and set the steam release handle to the *Sealing* position. Press the *Manual* button and cook for 25 minutes

When done; perform a quick pressure release and open the lid. Carefully remove the pan and set aside

Now press the *Saute* button. Add berries and pour in one cup of water and granulated stevia. Gently simmer for 5 - 6 minutes, stirring constantly

Finally, add agar powder and give it a good stir. Cook until the mixture thickens.

Pour the syrup over chilled cake and refrigerate for 2 hours before serving.

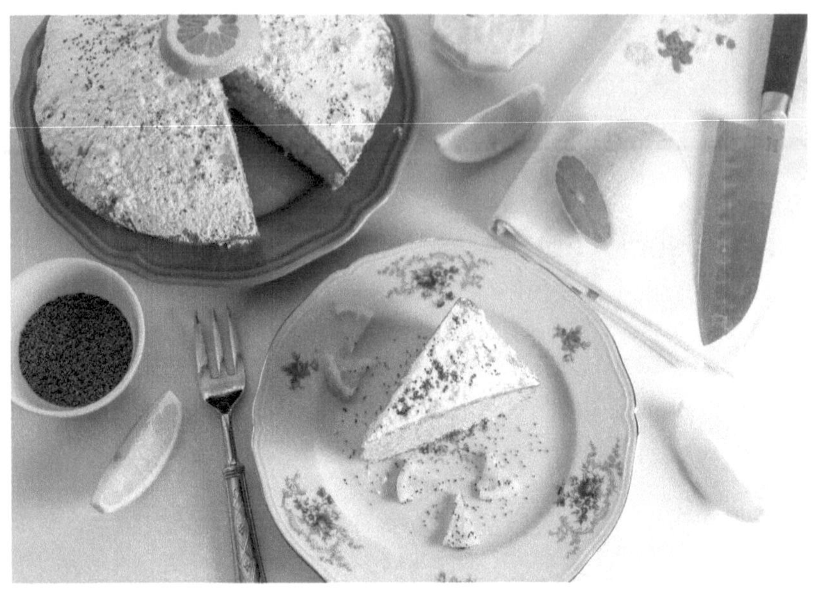

Choco Orange Muffins

Total time: 50 minutes

Ingredients

1/2 cup almond flour

5 large eggs

1/4 cup almonds; roughly chopped.

1 tbsp chia seeds

1 tbsp flaxseed meal

1/2 cup whole milk

1 tbsp butter

1 tbsp dark chocolate chips

1/2 tsp baking powder

1/4 tsp bicarbonate of soda

1/4 tsp cinnamon; ground

1 tsp orange extract

2 tsp stevia powder

Directions:

In a large mixing bowl, combine almond flour, almonds, chia seeds, flaxseed meal, baking powder, and bicarbonate of soda. Mix until well combined.

Add eggs, butter, milk, orange extract, stevia, and cinnamon. With a paddle attachment on, beat with a hand mixer for 2 - 3 minutes, or until well incorporated

Divide the mixture evenly between greased silicone muffin molds. Tuck in the chocolate chips and set aside

Plug in the instant pot and set the trivet on the bottom. Place the molds on top and close the lid. Adjust the steam release handle and press the *Manual* button. Set the timer for 30 minutes and cook on *High* pressure

When done; perform a quick pressure release and open the pot. Transfer the molds to a wire rack and let it cool to a room temperature

Rum Cheesecake

Total time: 40 minutes

Ingredients

2 cups almond flour

3 cups Mascarpone

4 large eggs; separated

1/4 cup coconut cream

1 cup plain Greek yogurt

2 - 3 drops stevia

2 tbsp almond butter

1/4 cup cocoa powder; unsweetened

1/4 cup swerve

3 tsp baking powder

1/2 tsp cinnamon powder

2 tsp rum extract

Directions:

Plug in the instant pot and position a trivet. Pour in one cup of water in the stainless-steel insert and set aside

Beat egg whites and swerve with a hand mixer until light foam appears. Add egg yolks, coconut cream, almond butter, baking powder, and cocoa powder, beating constantly

Finally, add almond flour and continue to beat until completely combined

Pour the mixture into lightly greased cake pan and cook for 15 minutes on the *Manual* mode

When done; perform a quick pressure release and open the lid. Remove the cake from the pan and cool for a while

Now combine Mascarpone and Greek yogurt. Add rum extract, cinnamon powder, and stevia. Using a hand mixer, mix well until completely combined

Pour the mixture over the crust and refrigerate for a couple of hours before slicing.

CONCLUSION

I hope that the chapters in this book have provided you with all the necessary information to help you achieve your health goals. After completing this book, you now know what the keto is and how to successfully stick to it using meal prepping methods. You can use any of the meal prepping ideas or even create some of your own that work best for you!

You can use any of the meal prepping ideas inside or even create some of your own that work best for you! But do remember, the keto diet is not a fad, but a lifestyle change to improve your body's condition. The objective of the keto diet is to convert healthy fats as the primary source of fuel rather than carbs to get through the day. Once you are in the metabolic state of ketosis, you will be more adept to lose weight and keep those bothersome pounds permanently off!

You now learn everything you need to live a healthy, lively, and satisfying lifestyle. You have the power now! I hope that you act now with the information presented in this book and use it to make your life a hundred times easier. You also have scrumptious keto-friendly recipes that can be prepared using the Instant Pot at your disposal. Your life will soon change for the better!